MEDICAL MARIJUANA

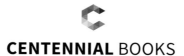

CENTENNIAL BOOKS

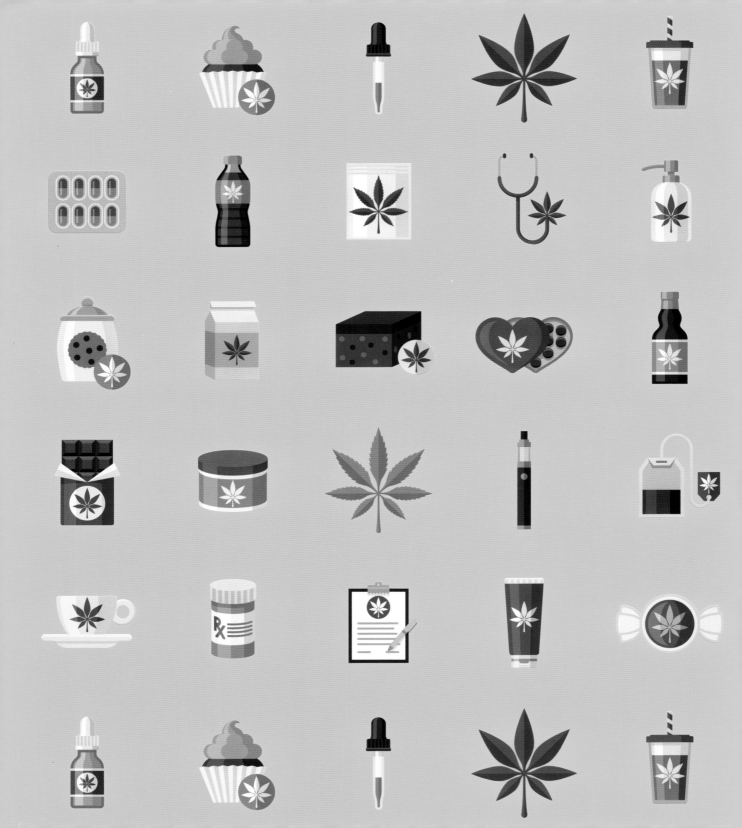

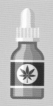
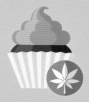
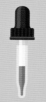
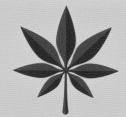
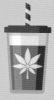

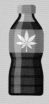

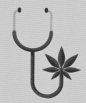

MEDICAL MARIJUANA

THE COMPLETE GUIDE

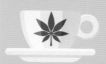

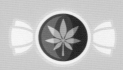

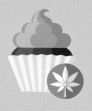

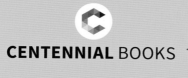
CENTENNIAL BOOKS

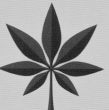
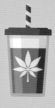

PART 1
GETTING STARTED

12 IS THIS THE FUTURE OF MEDICINE?

18 HOW IT REALLY WORKS

24 CRAZY FOR CBD

32 THE ABCS OF CBD PRODUCTS

36 DOSING WITH CANNABIS: A BEGINNER'S GUIDE

42 GIVING PHYSICIANS A NEW PRESCRIPTION

46 GETTING CARDED

50 PEACE STRAINS

56 ASK THE DOCTOR

PART 2
HEALING POWER

64 A-Z CANNABIS GUIDE TO HEALING

80 YOU ARE GETTING SLEEPY

86 GETTING BACK IN ACTION

92 CANCER & CANNABIS

96 COMFORT AFTER CHEMO

98 ENDING THE MISERY

102 OPTING OUT OF OPIOIDS

106 EASING THE TRAUMA

110 SENIOR MOMENTS

114 CBD IS THE CAT'S MEOW

118 HANDLE WITH CARE

122 IT'S ONLY NATURAL

126 POT CROCK?

PART 3
CANNABIS CHAMPIONS

132 POT'S PATRON SAINT: TOMMY CHONG

138 A TRUE BELIEVER: FRAN DRESCHER

142 CANNABIS CONVERT: DR. SANJAY GUPTA

148 COURTING CANNABIS: RICK BARRY

152 BUYING THE FARM: JIM BELUSHI

158 TAKING THE LEAD: DR. MEHMET OZ

166 A MOTHER'S FIGHT

176 OPPORTUNITY KNOX

180 SISTER ACT

186 INDEX

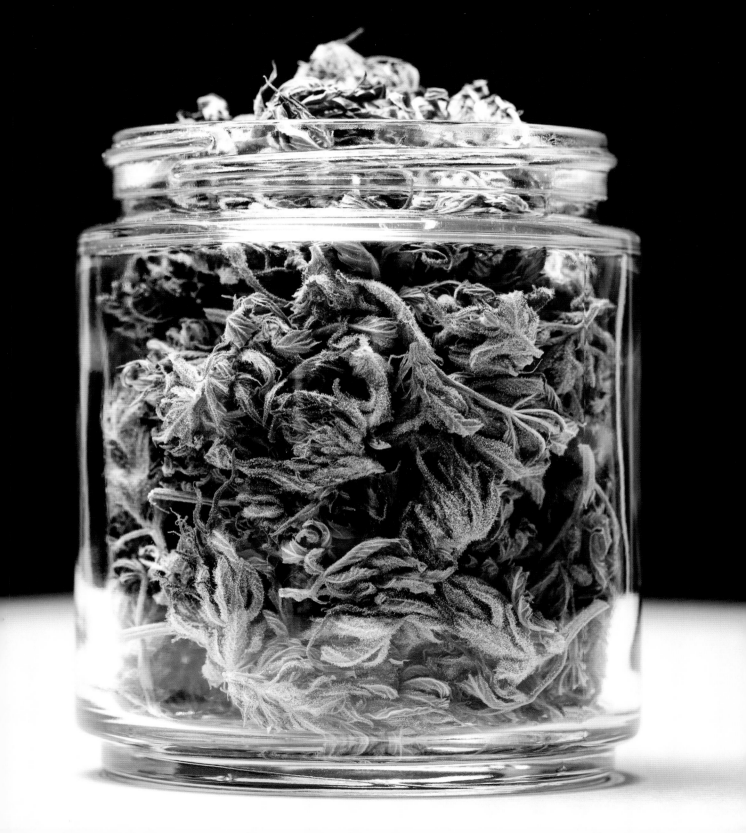

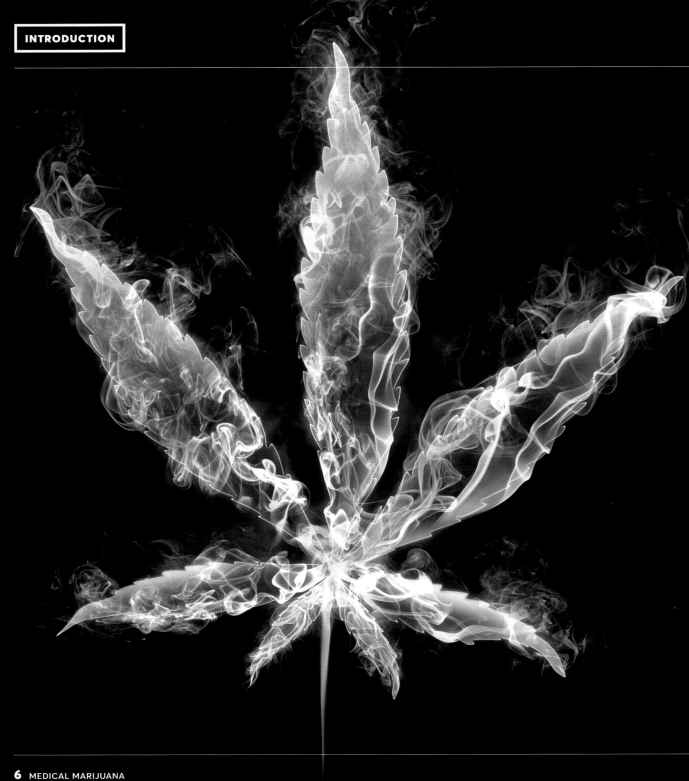

To be honest, it was a conversation topic that I never pictured bringing up with my mom. Talk about the grandkids? No problem. The weather? That's almost a given. My financial situation? It's bound to come up at some point. But marijuana? No way is that something a guy in his 50s ever imagines discussing with his 80-something mom. And yet these days, it's become a common occurrence for us.

Keep in mind that my mother is someone who used to be as anti-drug as anyone who came of age in the crew-cut clean 1950s and the hippie-hating 1960s. Hers was a generation that considered *Reefer Madness* to be a documentary rather than a propaganda film. Because this was her worldview, that naturally meant that I inherited it as well. Throughout my school years and beyond, I, too, considered cannabis use to be questionable at best. Still, as I began editing magazines about medical marijuana and my brother started using CBD for chronic back pain, my mom decided to confess something to me. She was eager to try CBD herself in order to see if it helped her never-ending arthritis pain.

At first, I was genuinely shocked by this revelation. However, I've since learned that my story is far from unique. Medical marijuana these days is kind of like

vitamins were back when I was growing up—an organic substance that once lived on the fringes of the medical world. Now, suddenly it feels like everyone has spoken to a parent or sibling or even a supermarket checkout clerk who swears that not only have they tried some form of medicinal marijuana, but they've also experienced incredible results. Whether it's the parent who has watched his or her child suffer from epileptic seizures, a cancer patient struggling through chemotherapy or an ex-athlete who can barely get out of bed because of joint pain, medical marijuana may be nothing short of a miracle.

It's should come as no surprise that a 2019 Pew Research Center found that 91 percent of U.S. adults believe that cannabis should be legal for some form of medical use. (Bear in mind that just 40 years ago only 12 percent of the country supported legalizin marijuana.) This result comes even though marijuana remains classified by the federal government as a Schedule 1 substance, meaning the feds view it as a drug with a high potential for abuse but without any legit medical purpose.

As a result of this pro-pot sentiment, 33 states had established some form of medical marijuana program as of the spring of 2020, and several more were edging closer to medicinal legalization. This escalating popularity has led experts to project that the U.S. market for cannabinoid-based medicines could easily hit $2 billion in 2020. Meanwhile, those meds now come in forms far beyond the traditional joint and bong we all remember from college, with relief arriving in everything from cannabis-laced candies and sodas to bath soaps, deodorants and sports drinks.

The more popular medical marijuana becomes, though, the more questions there are about exactly what it is and how it does what it does. And that is precisely what this book is all about. In the following pages, we'll explore the different components of medical marijuana and the physiology of how it works in the body. We'll also look at the wide variety of medical conditions that cannabis products can reportedly help: cancer, chronic pain, insomnia, anxiety, depression, anorexia, Crohn's disease, PTSD, glaucoma and many more. We'll break down the differences between the two essential elements taken from a cannabis plant, CBD (the nonintoxicating compound) and THC (the psychoactive compound responsible for the marijuana "high"). And, because so many people like my mom are using marijuana as medicine for the first time, we'll provide the basic information you'll need to know before making that initial, scary trip to your neighborhood dispensary.

None of this is intended to endorse the use of marijuana for medicinal (or any other) purposes. That's something everyone has to research and then decide for himself or herself after consulting with their health-care professional. Still, after living in the pharmaceutical-filled world that we've all now grown up in, it's nice to at least understand that there are potential alternatives out there that may not produce scary side effects such as addiction. Plus, if nothing else, getting to know more about this ever-expanding medical marijuana movement will provide one unexpected benefit. It'll give your mom something to talk with you about—besides the fact that you never seem to call her anymore.

—Craig Tomashoff

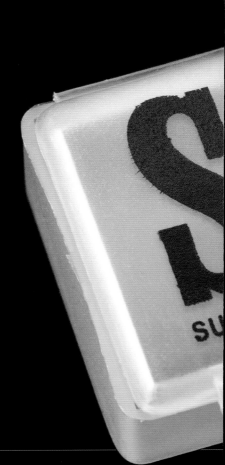

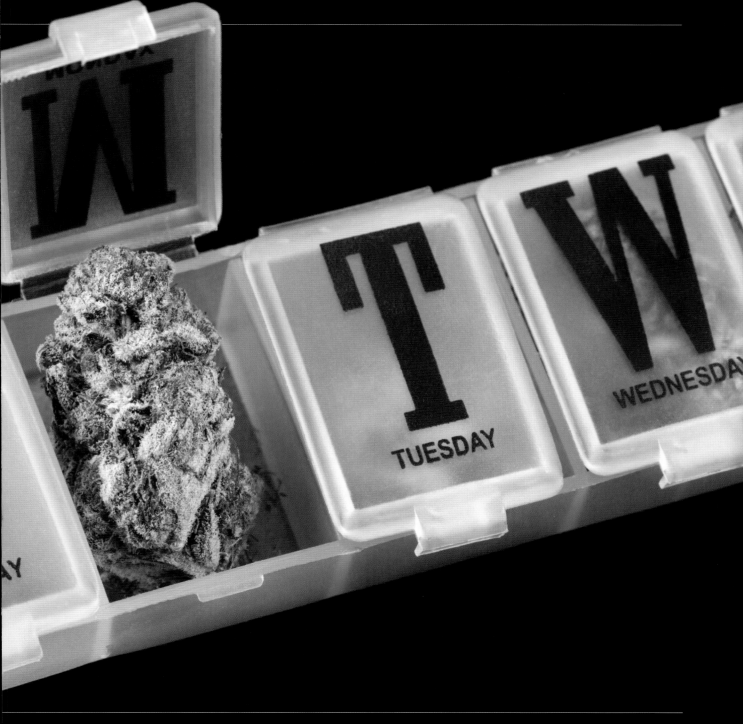

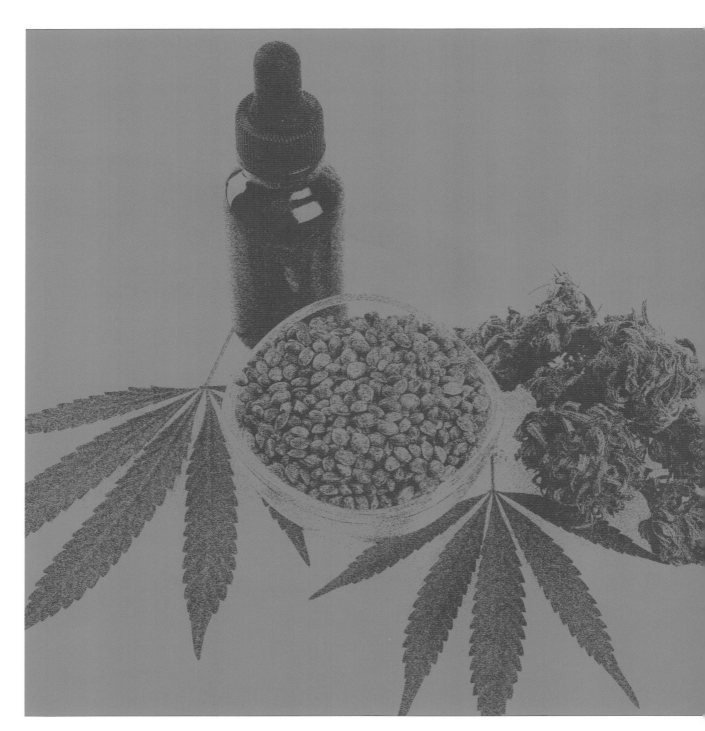

PART 1

GETTING STARTED

IS THIS THE FUTURE OF MEDICINE?

MEDICAL MARIJUANA IS GAINING POPULARITY, BUT NOT EVERYONE AGREES IT HELPS WHAT AILS US.

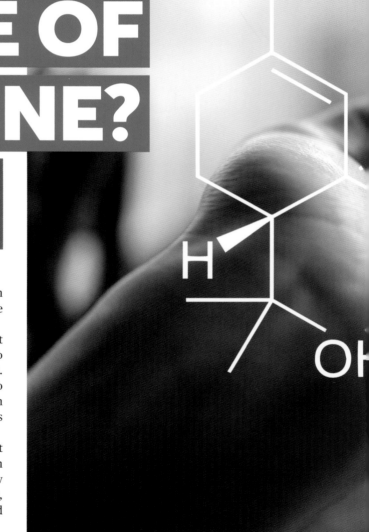

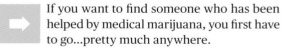 If you want to find someone who has been helped by medical marijuana, you first have to go...pretty much anywhere.

These days, no matter where you live or what you think of drug use, you know somebody who has used some form of cannabis to heal themselves. From cancer patients to children with epilepsy to soldiers coping with stress disorders to athletes with backaches, we live in an age where marijuana use is increasingly seen as a savior rather than a sin.

In late 2019, a Pew Research Center poll found that 91 percent of American voters support legalization either for medical or recreational use. There are now 46 states that authorize some form of medicinal use, and a survey by the Medical Marijuana Project found

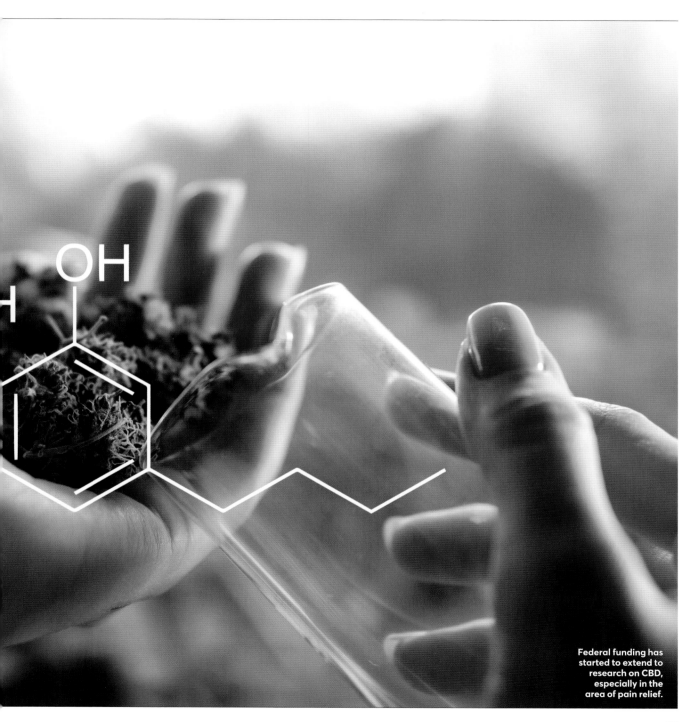

Federal funding has started to extend to research on CBD, especially in the area of pain relief.

that more than 2.3 million Americans are partaking of it legally. There's no doubt that the drive to legalize pot is spreading across the country and that medical use is what's behind the wheel.

"People have been told their whole lives that this is a drug, that it's a scary thing, that it leads to more dangerous things," explains Adie Rae, PhD, an award-winning researcher who has studied the effects of medical marijuana for more than a decade with assistance from the National Institute on Drug Abuse. "Some people have been convinced otherwise by the data on how much [cannabis] can help, but the majority have had to see it help a grandchild with epilepsy or a friend going through chemo before getting on board with it."

Not everyone, however, is a believer. For instance, there's Stuart Gitlow, MD, former president of the American Society of Addiction Medicine and now executive director of the Annenberg Physician Training Program in Addictive Disease. He believes "there's no such thing as medical marijuana. That's why there's no FDA approval, no prescribing and no medicine available." After 25 years as an addiction psychiatrist, he's still looking for hard science to back up claims that cannabis is a cure-all.

■ THE WARNINGS

Based on all he's seen and read throughout his career, Gitlow has come to believe one thing about the medical benefits of marijuana: There aren't any. There is, he believes, "no reason from a medical perspective to use it. If you're going to use it because you feel that you want to alter your brain's native state, and you don't care about the risks, be my guest. But for us to lie to people and tell them that there are significant benefits and minimal risks is not acceptable."

In particular, he is concerned about the risk of addiction. He concedes that only about 10 to 15 percent of people who use marijuana will end up using it addictively. Still, he's also convinced that shouldn't be justification to use it, because it's too soon to know if the drug is safe.

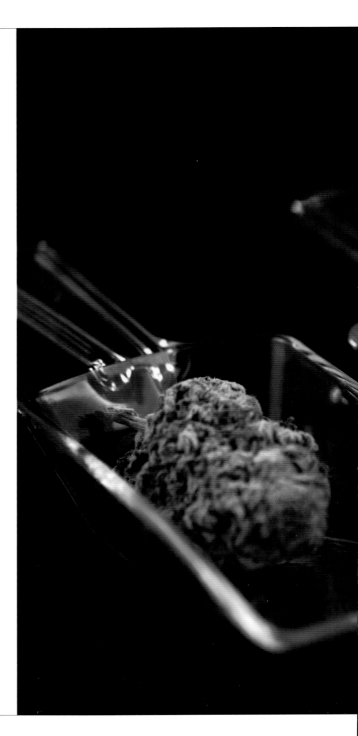

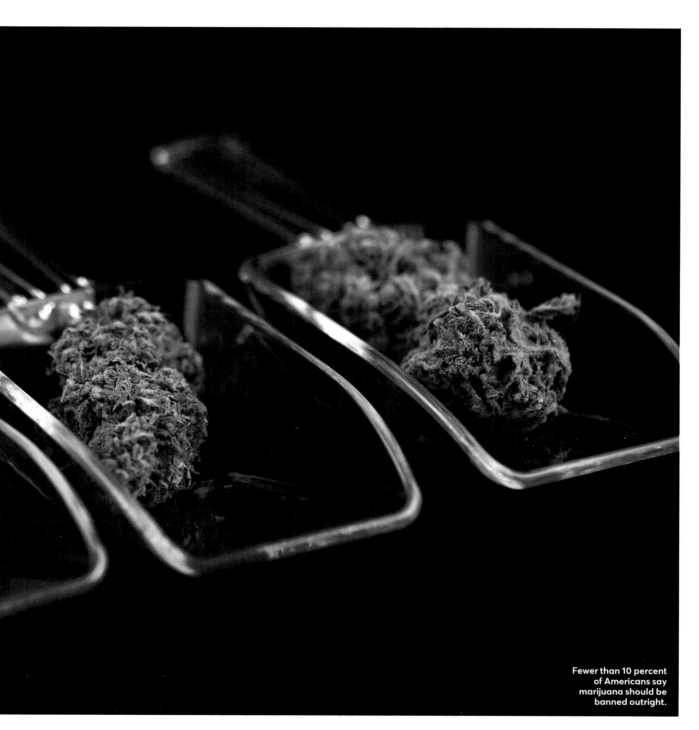

Fewer than 10 percent of Americans say marijuana should be banned outright.

"That means the vast majority of people can use it once in a while and have no significant downside. That's true in a car too...I can drive without a seat belt and the overwhelming likelihood is that I will never be hurt as a result," Gitlow explains. "But we mandate seat belts to protect the minority who would get hurt. Similarly, we need to protect the minority of people who would end up addicted to marijuana by having limitations on widespread use. We have such limitations now. Why would we change that?"

■ THE USES

Well, according to Rae, it's because the medical benefits of cannabis far outweigh any potential dangers. That's because of something all our bodies rely on: the endocannabinoid system (ECS). It plays a part in things like how we eat, sleep and stress out. Neurotransmitters are released in the brain that influence memory, movement, pleasure and countless other functions, and the ECS watches over it all.

"Think of neurotransmitters in your brain as being like kids trying to cross the street when school's out," says Rae. "The endocannabinoid system is the crossing guard trying to get the kids across but at the right time and the right rate. It's about volume control."

There are, she adds, "countless answers as to how [cannabis] restores biological processes, aids sleep and many other things." Her years of researching convinced her cannabis can do a better job of relieving pain and inflammation than any opioid. "The single greatest public health impact cannabis could have is to eliminate our dependence on opioids," explains Rae. "In states with medical cannabis laws, there are 25 percent fewer opioid overdoses. When patients are given access to cannabis, they will, on average, reduce opioid use by half. With pharmaceutical drugs, the side effects are often more unbearable than the pain. Cannabis is less toxic with fewer side effects."

■ THE EFFECTS

Even its most ardent supporters won't say that medical marijuana is a cure for everything that ails you.

However, they can all offer up countless anecdotes about how cannabis can provide relief to make life worth living again.

For instance, Rae has worked with a retired Missouri police officer who saw her husband die in the line of duty. That resulted in such severe PTSD that she flies to Seattle once a month to visit one of the legal dispensaries there. She buys some edible medical marijuana, returns to her hotel room where she takes it, sleeps for 10 straight hours for the first time all month, and then flies home.

Then there's the story of young Coltyn Turner, who has also inspired Rae's work. Coltyn is an Illinois boy who was diagnosed with Crohn's disease at age 11. Doctors tried all kinds of medications like Endacort and Humera to heal him and, at one point, suggested removing 22 inches of his diseased bowels. Unwilling to put her son through that, Wendy Turner researched medical marijuana. She found a caregiver in Colorado, and she sent her husband and Coltyn to experiment with using cannabis oils and brownies.

"A couple days into the brownie situation, my husband called to say he and Coltyn had taken a trip up to the mountains just to get out and escape cabin fever," Wendy says. "He told me Coltyn was throwing snowballs and running around. A couple weeks before, he'd been in a wheelchair and hadn't run in three years." (For more on Coltyn's story, turn to page 170.)

However, as far as opponents like Gitlow are concerned, these are ultimately just stories and not science. "I'm not particularly interested in anecdotal stories. That's not science," he explains. "If we approved medicines on the basis of anecdotes, we would be back to the age of quackery with the sales of mercury and silver-based products that have great danger and no significant value, but which anecdotally worked for some folks. If I have knee pain and you strike me in the head with a hammer, I am likely to say that my knee pain has dissipated. That doesn't mean my knee is better. It doesn't mean we should hit everyone who has knee pain in the head with hammers."

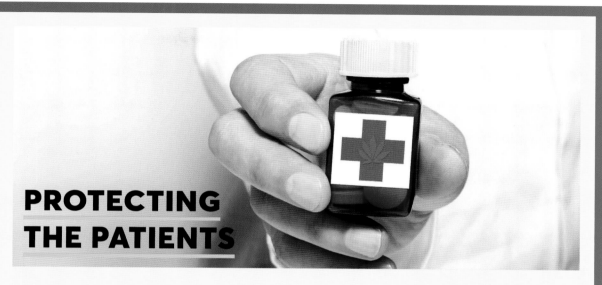

PROTECTING
THE PATIENTS

Despite concerns of scientists like psychiatrist Stuart Gitlow, medical marijuana seems to be catching on primarily because it doesn't seem so, well, "medical." To many, it's more like relying on an aloe vera plant for a sunburn, echinacea for colds or peppermint for a stomachache. It's a cure that comes from nature rather than a laboratory. When looked at in that context, medical cannabis is "changing the way we approach medicine in this country," according to Steph Sherer, executive director of Americans for Safe Access (ASA).

The ASA is the nation's largest member-based organization of patients, medical professionals, scientists and concerned citizens promoting the safe and legal use of medical marijuana. Sherer says she's encouraged at how far the country has come since California became the first state to authorize medicinal cannabis use in 1996, but she also realizes there is a long way to go.

"There's always a chance we could slip backward—and when I look at the population that needs cannabis, we're very far away from where we need to be," says Sherer, adding that ASA has been working on a campaign it has dubbed "End Pain, Not Lives " that tries to let the public know medical cannabis can be a tool in coping with the opioid crisis.

"It's not just saying you won't go to jail for using, but really making sure people know what it can do. We want to create an atmosphere where, upon diagnosis of a problem, doctors and patients automatically see this as an option to help. And that means not only creating a legal framework for the constant fight at the state and federal level but creating safety protocols for doing the research."

ASA has created what Sherer terms a "progress chart" to help potential patients determine if cannabis is an option:

■ Does the patient's state have a cannabis-use law?
■ Does it include cannabis use for pain (several states still don't)?
■ Does the patient's doctor know about these laws?
■ Does their hospital or hospice allow for medical cannabis use?
■ Can the patient afford a medical-use ID card?
■ Does the program allow people to have access fast enough?
■ Are there access centers near the patient?

HOW IT REALLY WORKS

A GUIDE TO THE WAYS MARIJUANA DOES WHAT IT DOES INSIDE THE BODY.

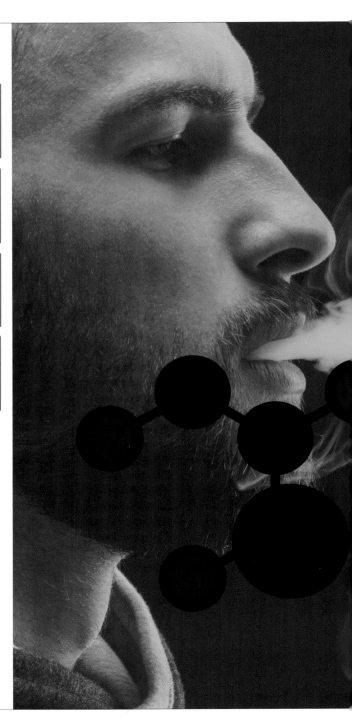

Nobody knows exactly when humans first discovered the intoxicating properties of cannabis. The current best estimate comes from a 2008 discovery in the Gobi Desert of an ancient burial site, which included a stash of high-THC weed that dates back to around 2700 B.C. What we do have a better handle on, though, is exactly how cannabis and its phytocannabinoids (cannabinoids from the plant) affect the mind and body.

Scientists have known for decades about the endocannabinoid system and that our bodies produce something called "endocannabinoids," which minimize pain, inflammation, stress and other

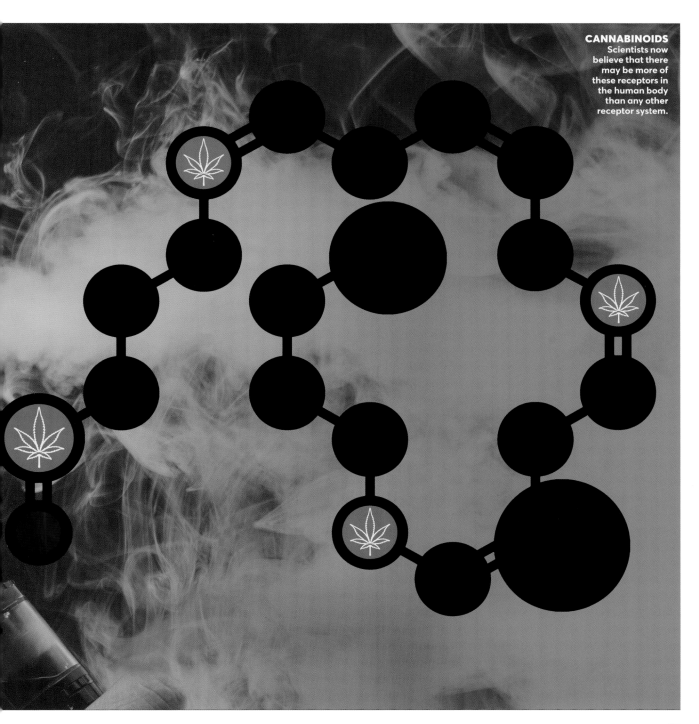

CANNABINOIDS
Scientists now
believe that there
may be more of
these receptors in
the human body
than any other
receptor system.

negative conditions; they also have known that cannabis's phytocannabinoids mimic the body's natural endocannabinoids. But it wasn't until researchers isolated the first cannabinoid receptor, CB1, and then the CB2 receptor, that they started to map out the endocannabinoid system (ECS). These discoveries led us to understand, thousands of years after people started getting high, how the body's endocannabinoid system works.

■ IT'S ALL ABOUT THE ECS

If we didn't have the endocannabinoid system, the system in our body that interacts with THC and CBD, we wouldn't get high or receive any of the therapeutic benefits from cannabis. Our body produces its own cannabinoids, called endocannabinoids; they keep our body in balance and act as "messengers" to tell it when to start and stop biological processes. Our cannabinoid receptors, together with these endocannabinoids, make up our ECS. So while our ECS responds to cannabis's phytocannabinoids, it's our endocannabinoids and the ECS that regulate important body functions like sleep, appetite, pleasure, pain and motor skills.

Named for the plant known as cannabis sativa, the ECS has multiple tasks, but it is primarily "responsible for maintaining balance in all of our human functions," explains neurologist Andrew Medvedovsky, the founder of New Jersey Alternative Medicine. The ECS is made up of three components: cannabinoid receptors (either CB1 or CB2), endocannabinoids ("messenger" molecules that bind to the receptors) and enzymes that break down the endocannabinoids.

This network of cannabinoid receptors, found throughout the body, binds not only with the endocannabinoids our bodies secrete naturally but also with the phytocannabinoids found in marijuana.

"In order for a compound to have an effect on the neurological system of the body, there has to be a receptor for it to interact with," explains Katie Stem, co-founder of Peak Extracts, the first adult-use edibles

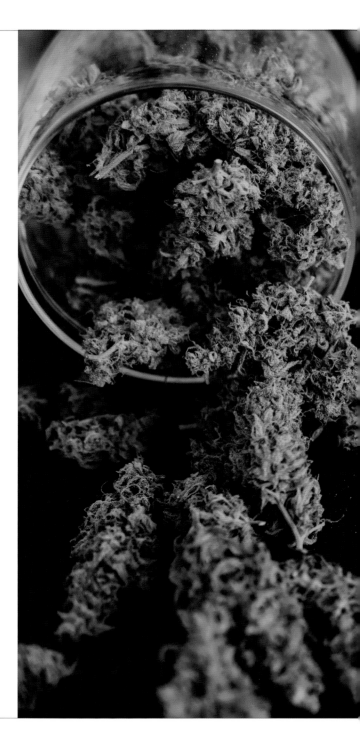

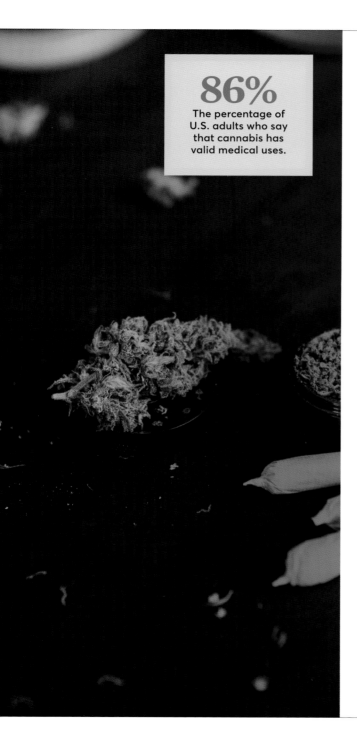

producer in Oregon. "One simple way to think about the receptors and the compounds that work with them is as a lock and key."

In other words, in the ECS system, if receptors are the lock, the cannabinoids are the key.

■ FINDING YOUR BLISS (OR NOT)

It turns out that THC, a psychoactive and intoxicating phytocannabinoid in marijuana, binds with the same receptors–CB1–as the endocannabinoid called anandamide, whose name is taken from "ananda," the Sanskrit word for bliss. Without these receptors, you can't get high. CB1 receptors are located in the central nervous system, with an abundance of receptors in the areas of the brain responsible for mental and physiological processes including memory, higher cognition, motor coordination, appetite and emotions. The ECS' CB2 receptors–which won't get you high–are found in the peripheral nervous system, the digestive system and in the immune system.

"THC is psychoactive and intoxicating, but CBD, while psychoactive–it interacts with the brain–isn't intoxicating," explains Stem. Although CBD may have less direct interaction with the body's cannabinoid receptors, it can still block the receptors, preventing one from getting too high.

"CBD modulates the activity of these receptors and THC," explains Medvedovsky. "Think of this like a pizza. What is the perfect pizza? It has perfect crust, just enough sauce and cheese. Cannabis is a perfect plant. If you only take the THC, you're just eating the cheese. It's good in small amounts but too much and you'll get sick. If you just eat the crust and the sauce, you're just having CBD–it will fill you up but it's not going to give you the complete effect. You need both. THC and CBD are partners; they work together."

So exactly how does weed work in the body? After it's been smoked or ingested, the THC and CBD move throughout the body in the bloodstream, heading to the CB1 and CB2 receptors. Once there, the THC

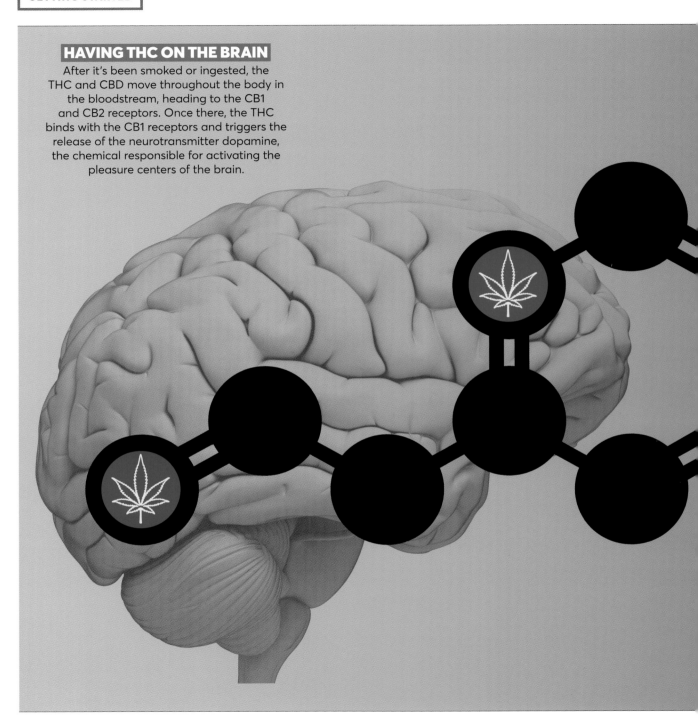

HAVING THC ON THE BRAIN

After it's been smoked or ingested, the THC and CBD move throughout the body in the bloodstream, heading to the CB1 and CB2 receptors. Once there, the THC binds with the CB1 receptors and triggers the release of the neurotransmitter dopamine, the chemical responsible for activating the pleasure centers of the brain.

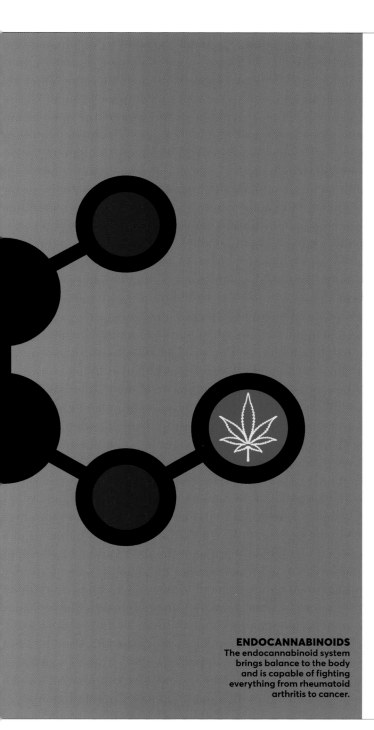

ENDOCANNABINOIDS
The endocannabinoid system brings balance to the body and is capable of fighting everything from rheumatoid arthritis to cancer.

We should legalize medical marijuana. We should do it nationally. And we should do it now."

DR. SANJAY GUPTA, ON CNN

binds with the CB1 receptors and triggers the release of the neurotransmitter dopamine, the chemical responsible for activating the pleasure centers of the brain. THC doesn't act on dopamine directly but helps the brain to get the message out to bump up production. For most people, this creates a sense of euphoria and well-being. As THC binds to the CB1 receptors, it becomes more difficult for the endocannabinoids to facilitate communication between cells. CBD, while it doesn't get you high, does inhibit enzymes from breaking down anandamide, the body's own bliss cannabinoid.

Even now, researchers admit we don't know everything about how cannabis interacts with the body. "It's a complex process; we don't understand all of the details yet. But cannabis is safe for generally healthy people," explains neuroscientist Adie Rae, PhD. "If you look at how long people have been using cannabis, we can say clinical trials of cannabis were done 5,000 years ago in China!"

CRAZY FOR CBD

FROM BATH SALTS TO PET TREATS, THE CANNABIS COMPOUND IS PURPORTED TO BE A VIRTUAL CURE-ALL TO HELP REDUCE PAIN, IMPROVE SLEEP, BOOST MOOD AND MORE. WE'RE HERE TO HELP YOU FIGURE OUT WHAT'S REAL.

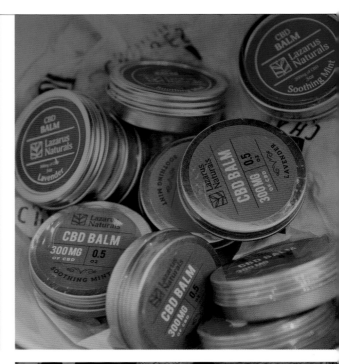

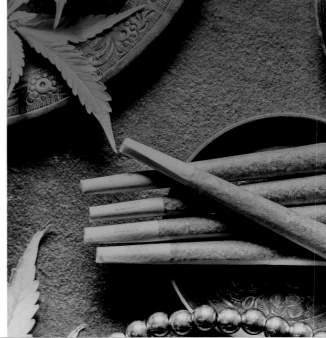

Google "CBD products" and you get more than 200 million results. It seems like overnight CBD oils, capsules, creams, tinctures, edibles and sprays are literally everywhere. And they're not just online: mainstay retailers like Walgreens and Bed, Bath & Beyond are selling these cannabis-derived products, too. You can even find CBD vape pens at gas stations.

Said to cure a lot of what ails us, from pain and depression to insomnia and sexual dysfunction, CBD–which is shorthand for the compound cannabidiol–has gone from a fringe fascination to a mainstream marvel. Sales in 2019 topped $5 billion, a whopping 706 percent increase over 2018, according to cannabis market research firm the Brightfield Group. By 2022, sales could reach $23 billion in the U.S. alone. What in the name of Cheech & Chong is going on?

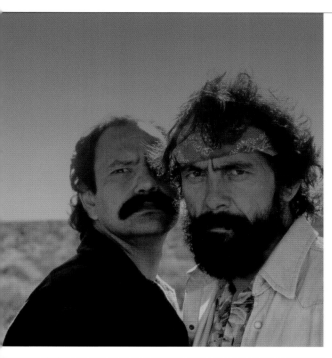

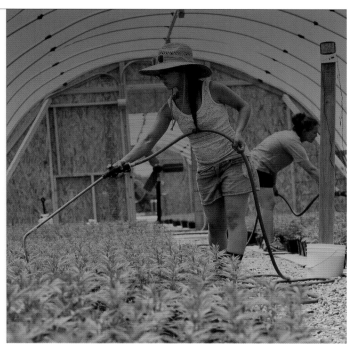

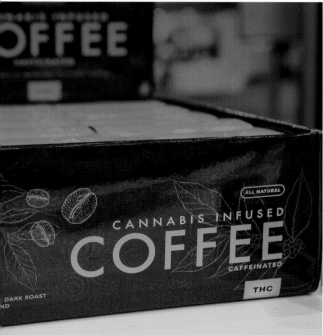

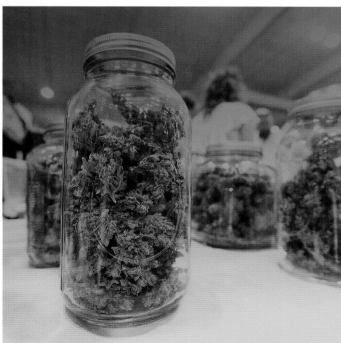

1 THE HEMP REVOLUTION

For starters, humans love a good cure-all. But the real CBD rush began with the legalization of hemp under the 2018 Farm Bill, as well as the sale of products made from it nationwide. Hemp, a variety of cannabis, can be used to produce CBD, provided it doesn't contain more than 0.3 percent of tetrahydrocannabinol (THC), the chemical compound that gets users "high" and is found more abundantly in hemp's cousin, marijuana.

"For a long time, we've been trying to convince people to stop going into a dispensary and buying the most grams of THC for their dollar, and instead buy the most enjoyable experience for their dollar—and lo and behold, here comes hemp," explains Adie Rae, PhD, an assistant scientist with Legacy Research Institute and a leading cannabis researcher. "It's this unexpected gift. We were trying to convince people not to drink moonshine, and then, boom, Bud Light shows up on the market. I really welcome it. It's a very exciting time where we're going to see really interesting phytochemically diverse types of hemp being introduced."

Studies have produced some evidence of CBD's beneficial effects, including strong anti-inflammatory and antioxidant components. CBD has also been shown to facilitate positive mood states and reduce stress by alleviating cortisol in the body, notes Rae. "We also know that it has a massive margin of safety," she says. "There may be some pretty substantial placebo effects happening with it–as with any new drug–but from my perspective, that's great. This is a drug that does absolutely nothing except make people feel better." In fact, many people even dispute using the word "drug" in reference to cannabidiol and prefer to think of hemp-based CBD as one would a vitamin or supplement.

2 FORM AND FUNCTION

CBD may work because it can go hand in hand with our own physiology. The human body manufactures its own cannabinoids (CB) that help maintain a baseline of health for many

Horticulture 101

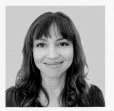

Adie Rae, PhD

Hemp and marijuana are two different species of the Cannabis sativa plant. Both produce cannabidiol (CBD), but differ in their concentration of THC (tetrahydrocannabinol). While THC in marijuana can exceed 15 percent, the amount in legalized hemp is supposed to be 0.3 percent or less. In other words, no matter how much hemp-derived CBD you use, you really shouldn't feel any euphoric effects.

To extract CBD oil from cannabis flowers, many manufacturers use some kind of solvent, like propane or butane, which is then removed, although trace amounts can remain. CO_2 extraction is also popular. "My favorite method is to flash-freeze the flower and then the little structures [resin glands] that hold all of that oil become very brittle and fall right off with a little agitation," says Rae, who is also a teacher at Washington University in St. Louis. "There's no solvent, and it's not labor-intensive at all. It's a very pure product."

physiological and neurological functions. However, elements like stress, a poor diet and illness can throw our systems out of whack. That's where CBD comes in. The compound can positively interact with the CB

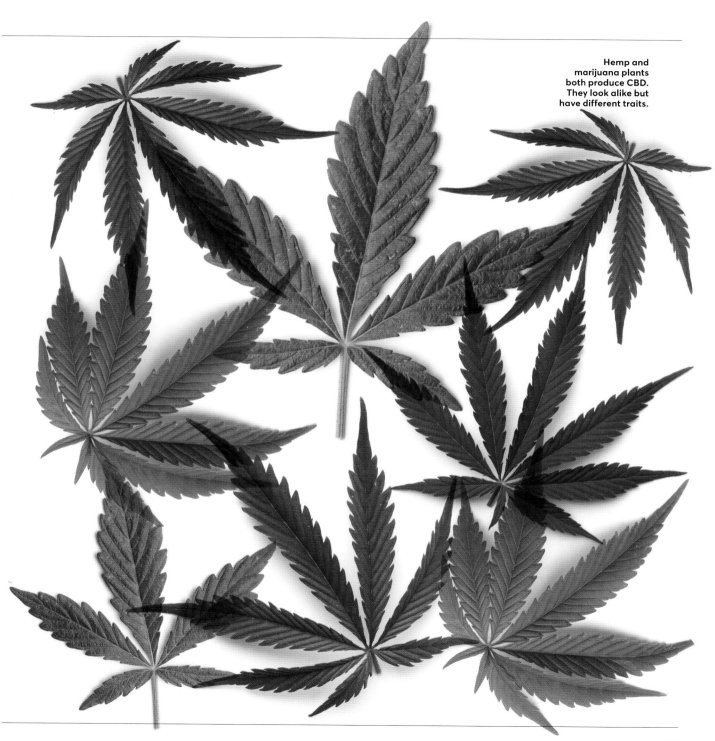

Hemp and marijuana plants both produce CBD. They look alike but have different traits.

receptors in the body, helping to correct imbalances in everything from our brains to our internal organs. The receptors, CB1 and CB2, sit on cell surfaces and act like guards. CB1 receptors are essential for a healthy functioning brain and central nervous systems, while CB2 receptors help moderate our immune response to microorganisms, particularly with regard to inflammation. And cannabinoids have the secret password to unleash a downstream effect that will rapidly impact a variety of bodily functions.

3 MEDICAL BENEFITS

You can now easily order CBD online, purchase it locally at the drugstore (including most major national chains) or at the new CBD store that opened in your neighborhood. But should you? Our answer is yes. Some critics contend that the industry is riddled with issues, and while there is some truth to that, as with many new industries norms are being established and hemp-based CBD is generally seen as safe, with few side effects and many positive benefits. The same day that Congress passed the Farm Bill on December 12, 2018, the Food and Drug Administration (FDA), which has the authority to regulate products containing cannabis or cannabis-derived compounds, expressed concern over the number of CBD products on the market that claim to have therapeutic benefits. According to the FDA, any product that purports to have a health claim must first be approved by the agency. And so far, the FDA has approved only one pharmaceutical drug containing CBD—Epidiolex, which was created for children who have one of two rare, severe forms of epilepsy: Lennox-Gastaut syndrome and Dravet syndrome.

Fortunately, the Farm Bill has also made it much easier to conduct research on products that were once banned. There is a wide variety of studies currently underway to evaluate CBD's ability to alleviate issues such as anxiety or post-traumatic stress disorder (PTSD), or to help with substance abuse and tobacco cessation. Funding from the National Institutes of Health for CBD studies shot up from virtually zero in 2014 to about $16 million in 2018. And in September 2019, the NIH announced nine new research awards totaling about $3 million earmarked to investigate some of the pain-relieving properties of CBD and other cannabinoids and terpenes.

Many companies who make hemp-based CBD follow the guidelines applied to the vitamins and supplements industry. Just as there are drugs that doctors prescribe and that the FDA regulates, there is a parallel market to treat ailments using natural remedies. CBD is widely accepted to ease pain, relieve anxiety and help people sleep. So just as you might take melatonin to fall asleep at night, CBD has many of the same benefits. The consensus is that over time more standards will be adopted, which we think is a good thing for consumers—and like with any product, you may have to experiment with brands, doses and consumption methods to find what works best for you. Many doctors and family physicians are educating themselves on the space, so whether it's this book, websites, magazines, medical professionals or friends, there are lots of places to learn more.

4 DOSING ADVICE

If the studies confirm the anecdotal evidence of CBD's beneficial effects, there are two other issues to consider: How much CBD are you really getting in a product, and what is the best way to consume it?

It's very difficult for consumers to know if products are accurately labeled, because there are no third-party laboratory testing requirements with CBD as there are with marijuana in legalized states. A 2017 Penn Medicine study found that only 30 percent of the 84 CBD extracts that were bought online contained an actual CBD content that was within 10 percent of the amount that was listed on the product label. A number of the products also contained a significant amount more THC than the 0.3 percent or less that legalized

Consumption Junction

Here's a look at the different ways to consume CBD. Studies suggest a full-spectrum CBD, rather than an isolate, is more effective because of the better absorption rates of products in their natural form (the so-called entourage effect), but if having a minute amount of THC in your system is an issue for work or other reasons, then an isolate is a safer bet.

NASAL SPRAYS
Quick-acting, with high bioavailability, like pre-rolls.

TOPICALS
Used for site-specific discomfort like knee pain; has very low bioavailability (the absorption rate into the bloodstream).

PRE-ROLLS
High bioavailability rates—between 34 and 46 percent. However, smoke of any kind is carcinogenic and harmful to your lungs.

DRY-HERB VAPING
The whole plant product without any of the dangers of oil-based vaping or pre-roll combustion. Similar bioavailability to pre-rolls.

TINCTURES
An oil that is placed under the tongue for a few minutes and absorbed directly into the bloodstream through the sublingual gland. Bioavailability rates range between 12 and 25 percent.

OIL VAPING
High bioavailability—but with all of the issues surrounding the technology (due to synthetic marijuana and additives like vitamin E acetate), probably not the best option until the smoke clears.

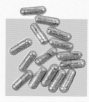

CAPSULE/PILL/GUMMY
A good way to experiment with how CBD works in your system, but be aware that the bioavailability is very low, between 4 and 20 percent, according to a 2007 National Institutes of Health study.

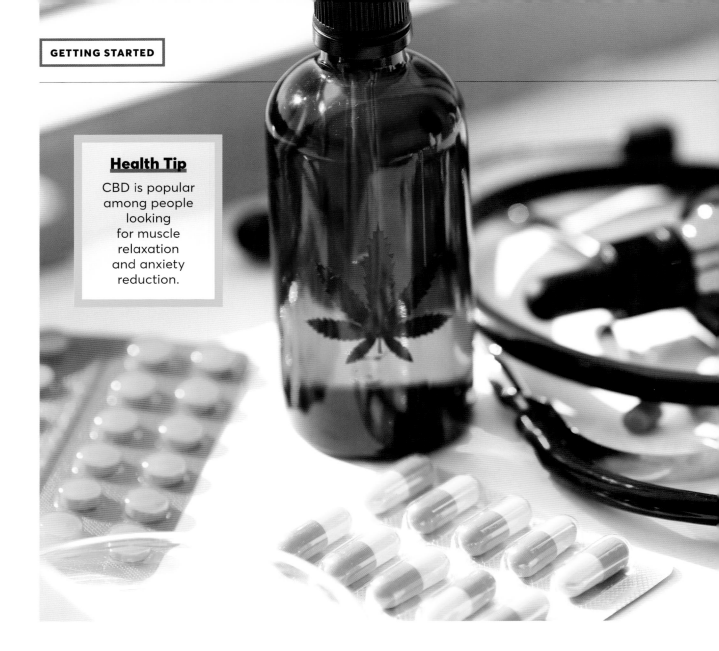

Health Tip

CBD is popular among people looking for muscle relaxation and anxiety reduction.

hemp is supposed to have. Pesticide contamination in the products is also a concern.

And then there's the consumption conundrum. Are you actually getting your money's worth? Quality CBD isn't cheap: A 750 mg bottle of 30 capsules from a top brand goes for around $90. "One huge problem with CBD is that it has incredibly low oral bioavailability," notes Rae. Scientists note that just 5 percent of a capsule's contents makes it through your liver and into your bloodstream. "But if you're inhaling CBD through a whole plant vaporizer, for instance, roughly 50 to 70 percent makes it into your bloodstream."

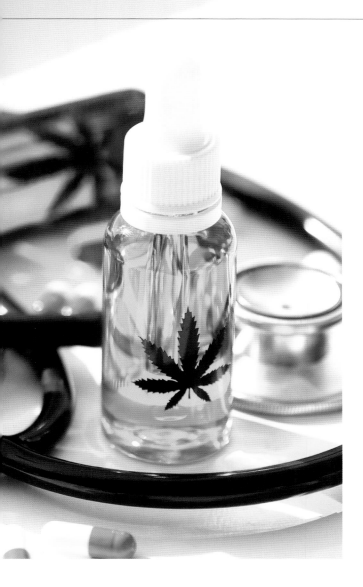

suspect online sites or stores in California, Florida, Maryland and South Carolina found that one-third of the products contained synthetic marijuana.

The most popular way to consume CBD oil is through a tincture of oil placed under the tongue, but most people don't leave it there nearly long enough, says Rae. A tincture dose needs to stay under the tongue for four minutes—a lot longer than the 10 to 30 seconds that is common practice. And the amount that winds up in your system varies wildly due to the different absorption rates for the various oils it's suspended in (which include coconut, almond, jojoba, olive and pure hemp).

5 ON THE MARKET

So, what's a savvy consumer to do? Start by looking for companies that display their third-party laboratory results on their website and shop for a broad-spectrum CBD, which seems to be more effective than an isolate or pure CBD product because of its suite of other cannabis molecules. Studies by Tikun Olam, a leading cannabis research firm, show that CBD-rich products with some THC and other compounds from the plant work better than pure CBD.

"I am very much in the ensemble camp," says Rae. "We know from 5,000 years ago starting in China that consumption of the whole plant is a safe and effective therapy and that there's no reason to deviate from that safety and efficacy."

Your correct dosage depends on your needs, chemistry and the type of product. If you live in a state where marijuana is legal, consider experimenting with a full-spectrum CBD that has more than 0.3 THC in it, especially if you suffer from chronic pain or insomnia.

The key is to experiment and patiently figure out what works with the help of some scientific note-taking in the process. Doing so might just unlock that magic bullet we've all been looking for and make CBD more than just a passing fad. "Cannabis has been an incredibly useful plant for millennia," says Rae. "It's high time, no pun intended, that we have access to it."

Dry-herb vaporization, which "bakes" finely ground flower, doesn't have any of the risks associated with the vaping scare going on, which seems partially due to synthetic marijuana, according to recent investigations by the Centers for Disease Control. Laboratory tests on 30 different CBD oil cartridges purchased from

THE ABCS OF CBD PRODUCTS

A LEADING CBD EXPERT OUTLINES THE TOP SEVEN THINGS TO BE WARY OF WHEN BUYING CBD FOR THE FIRST TIME.

CBD is undeniably having a moment, and for good reason: Many CBD users swear by the cannabinoid's ability to ease everything from anxiety to achy muscles. Perhaps you're curious about CBD, but don't quite know where to start. The array of CBD products available to the consumer right now is incredibly varied—and it can be expensive, so it's a good idea to fully inform yourself before setting out on a shopping spree. We asked Zoe Sigman, program director at the California-based nonprofit Project CBD, to provide some important tips on what consumers should look for when they are buying CBD for the first time.

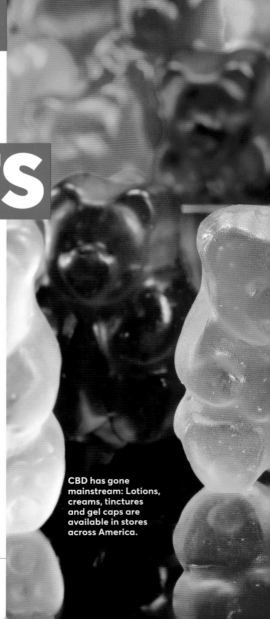

CBD has gone mainstream: Lotions, creams, tinctures and gel caps are available in stores across America.

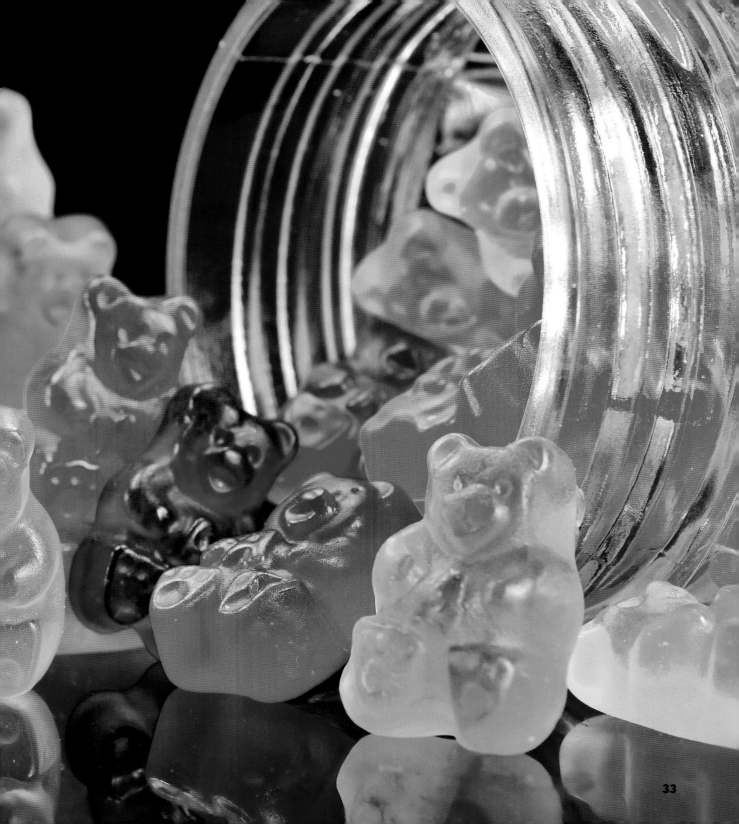

1

DO YOUR HOMEWORK

CBD currently has a large and unregulated market in the United States. This means that the quality of products available can run the gamut. "The onus is on the consumer to do their due diligence," says Sigman. "Be willing to communicate with the makers of the product. Are they using flower that was grown in sustainable ways, without the use of pesticides? If they are using really high-quality flower, they're going to want to show it off."

2

BUY FROM THE RIGHT VENDORS

"In general, companies from states that have legalized cannabis are held to higher standards, because their states require it," Sigman explains. Because of this, it's often advisable to seek out products that originate in states like California or Oregon. If you're in a state with legalized cannabis, it's a good idea to ensure that you trust the dispensary you're buying from. Are the budtenders approachable and willing to talk things through with you? Do you see products on the shelves that have organic certifications? "Look for companies that have gone above and beyond

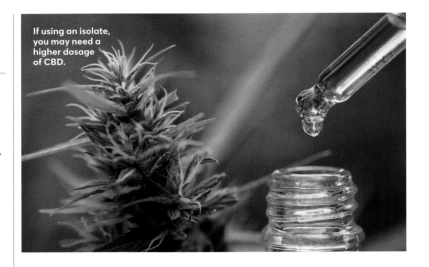

If using an isolate, you may need a higher dosage of CBD.

to work with a certification company to show that their work is high quality," Sigman adds.

3

DIAL IN ON YOUR DOSE

There is no one-size-fits-all CBD dose, and achieving the results you're looking for will require that you find what works for you and your body. One of the first things to consider is the difference between isolate and full-spectrum CBD. In this case, isolate refers to cannabidiol that's isolated from the plant's other cannabinoids. Full-spectrum oils, on the other hand, contain small amounts of THC. "People who are using pure CBD isolates might need to take a much higher dosage of CBD than if they're

taking something that contains a little THC or some of the other minor cannabinoids," Sigman notes. Figuring out what dose you should take will also require a little "guess and check" work. According to Sigman, 10 mg to 30 mg is a general ballpark dosage to start with for many people. "If you don't feel anything, don't be afraid to increase your dose. It's not a dangerous compound to ingest. There isn't a maximum dose."

4

LEARN TO LIKE LABELS

"Look for really clear labels that show the actual cannabinoid content, and have doses that are clearly indicated," she says. "Look for a tincture dropper that has demarcated lines that correlate to some kind of dosing info on the package. It's a really good way to keep track of how much you're taking and whether or not it's effective."

5

KNOW WHAT YOU WANT TO TREAT

Unlike THC, which is a psychotropic, CBD is not intoxicating, which is one reason noticing its effects may require some mindfulness. "The effects can be kind of subtle and mood-altering," Sigman says. For this reason, she advises new users to know what they want to treat, whether it's anxiety, pain, insomnia, PTSD or any one of the other ailments it's purported to help. This will allow you to check in after you've taken your first dose and see whether you notice any shift in how you feel. Then you can adjust your dose accordingly.

6

CHOOSE A CONSUMPTION METHOD THAT WORKS BEST FOR YOU

As you may have already noticed, there are quite a few delivery systems available when it comes to consuming CBD. Which method works best for you will depend on your personal preferences and the results you are hoping to achieve.

"Inhalation is the fastest method and has the shortest duration. It also has the highest bioavailability," says Sigman, referring to how effectively it gets into your bloodstream. "When you consume CBD by inhaling it, you're going to get a lot of bang for your buck." Edibles, on the other hand, have a much lower bioavailability and will take longer to kick in, but you will feel their effects longer. "They can take up to a few hours to take effect, so that's just something to be aware of. If you don't feel something after an hour, wait a little longer," she offers. Topicals used for muscle aches have zero bioavailability, so the benefits are more likely placebo. But she says they can be a "really approachable way for a lot of people to start thinking about cannabis."

7

KNOW YOUR CANNABIS

When shopping around for CBD, you will notice many products are derived from hemp, marijuana's cannabis cousin. Hemp products must contain less than 0.3 percent THC to be legal. Though it has traditionally been grown for fiber and seeds, many farmers are now breeding "craft hemp" specifically designed to emphasize CBD that can be full-spectrum. "Craft hemp has just as wonderful a chemical expression as something grown from cannabis," Sigman advises. If you're not happy with one product, she says, there are plenty more to choose from.

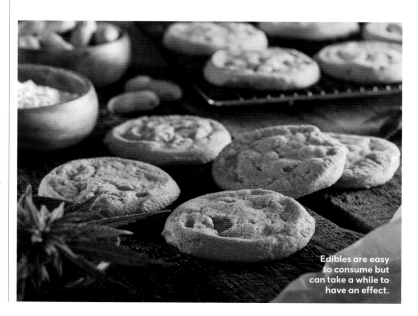

Edibles are easy to consume but can take a while to have an effect.

DOSING WITH CANNABIS: A BEGINNER'S GUIDE

PAIN? STRESS? INSOMNIA? HERE'S HOW TO USE MEDICAL CANNABIS TO TREAT ALL THREE CONDITIONS WITHOUT GETTING HIGH.

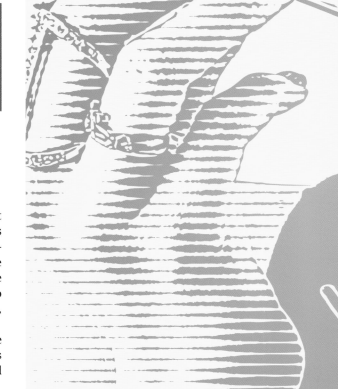

A few years ago, a nasty bout of gout left me with arthritis in my two large toes. This made walking painful, running excruciating and the inevitability of growing older ever more apparent. I'm a guy in midlife. I eat well, exercise consistently and spend a lot of time and money to keep my body from obsolescence. Needless to say, this malfunction did not make me happy.

A parade of doctors and specialists offered me Advil and Tylenol, but neither of these NSAIDs did much to relieve the pain. They're also linked

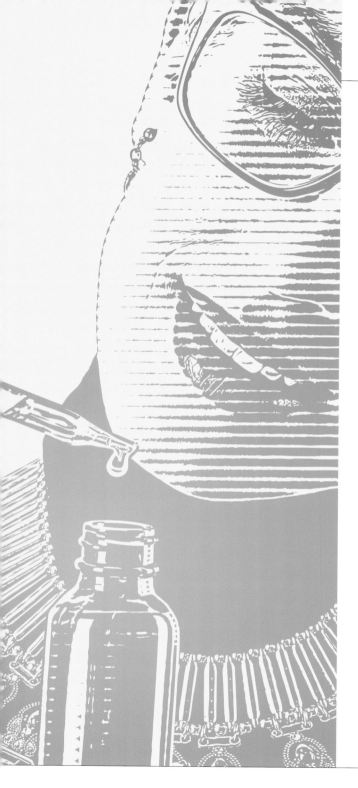

to a host of stomach-wrenching side effects, so I decided to experiment with medical cannabis. The only problem was finding a reliable guide to dosing. Also—and this is a big one—I'm a writer and a consultant, and the nature of my work doesn't allow me to be high.

After a lot of investigation and many hours spent interviewing scientists, cannabis physicians and researchers, I created medicalcannabismentor.com, the first online course for patients who want to use medical cannabis to treat three conditions—pain, insomnia and stress—without necessarily getting high. These are the most common ailments cannabis is used for and evidence shows that it works as well as—if not better than—off-the-shelf and prescription medications on the market. Here's a condensed version of what I've learned.

■ FIRST, THE BASICS

Medical cannabis is not simply a smoke-a-joint-and-get-so-high-you-forget-the-condition approach to healing. Nor is it a one-size-fits-all approach. It's about finding the lowest measurable dose of cannabinoids to get maximum relief for your particular metabolism.

Cannabis is a complex chemical factory of over 600 compounds. THC and CBD are the two most prevalent cannabinoids.

THC causes the high and feelings of euphoria. It also brings on side effects, which include temporary racing of the heart, interruption of short-term memory, loss of balance and paranoia. Some medical journals claim the high is also an "unwanted side effect." For some that's true, but for others it's a powerful medicine that also creates some euphoria—not necessarily such a bad thing.

The second most prevalent cannabinoid is CBD. Even though it was discovered at the same time as THC, this compound got little notice because it is not psychoactive. In past decades, scientists have discovered that CBD is a potent pain reliever and anti-inflammatory—20 times more powerful than aspirin and twice as powerful as hydrocortisone.

COMBINING THC WITH CBD HAS TWO BENEFITS:
For one, THC amplifies the therapeutic effects of CBD. In addition, CBD offsets the negative effects and mitigates the psychoactivity of THC, which makes it ideal for those of us who want to be functional while medicating.

The Medical Cannabis Mentor program starts all patients with pure CBD. Those who require more relief can then introduce THC in small doses, minimizing the side effects.

Like all botanical medicines, cannabis requires self-administration, which is nothing new even in allopathic medicine. Diabetics adjust their insulin depending on their blood sugar levels. Pain patients tinker constantly with the amount of gabapentin they take. The only difference is that cannabis is so much safer than any other drug.

The process of finding your optimal dose usually takes a few weeks. You'll get the best result if you allow 60 to 90 days to experiment with:

- The amount you use.
- The frequency with which you use it
  (twice a day, four times a day or more).
- The method you choose to get it into your body.

▦ METHODS OF MEDICATING

There are at least four methods of medicating with cannabis, all of which have their advantages and disadvantages. The methods you choose will depend on the conditions you are treating. In all cases, it's useful to keep a record of what you took, as well as how much and when. This will enable you to easily see what worked for which condition.

▦ INHALATION

Inhalation is the fastest way to get immediate relief, as cannabinoids are absorbed into the bloodstream within 10 to 15 seconds. Previously, medical professionals favored vaping to smoking, since it tends to be more convenient and efficient. However,

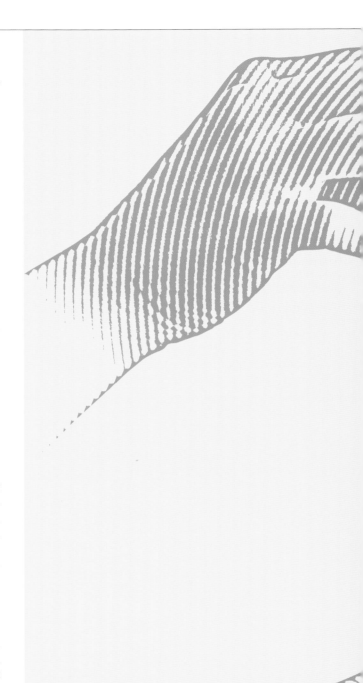

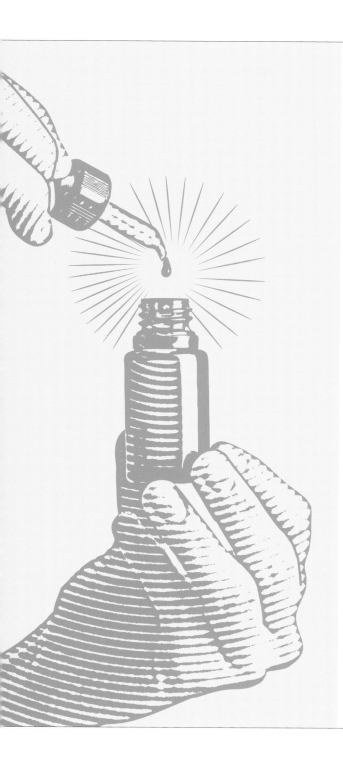

an outbreak of serious lung illnesses in 2019 led many to reconsider this method. The majority of vaping-related illnesses were traced by the Centers for Disease Control and Prevention (CDC) to vitamin E acetate, which was used to dilute the oils used in vaping. And most of the cases centered on THC and/or nicotine, not CBD specifically. Still, health experts are concerned that the mere act of heating solvents to high temperatures can be dangerous. So until more is known about vaping, you're best off steering clear of this method.

▬ TINCTURES

Tinctures are extracted cannabinoids mixed in alcohol or oil. Many medical providers see these as the future as they are easy to dose, relatively fast-acting, smoke-free and premixed in THC:CBD ratios, which makes finding the right blend for your condition easy. There are 4 types of tinctures:

1 PURE CBD
Not psychoactive
GOOD FOR Inflammation, anxiety, pain, relaxation

2 HIGH CBD:LOW THC
CBD:THC in ratios of 18:1 or above
Limited psychoactivity
GOOD FOR Pain relief (non-sedating), anti-inflammation, convulsing, anxiety, mood stabilizing

3 CBD:THC IN MORE EQUAL RATIOS
CBD:THC in ratios of 8:1, 4:1, 2:1, 1:1
Mild-moderate psychoactivity
GOOD FOR Pain relief, anti-inflammation, muscle relaxer, antidepressant, anxiety, nausea

4 HIGH THC:LOW CBD
Psychoactive
GOOD FOR Insomnia, nausea and vomiting, appetite stimulation, anti-anxiety, mood enhancer and muscle relaxer

Tinctures are also very versatile. They can be swallowed for long-lasting relief, swished in the

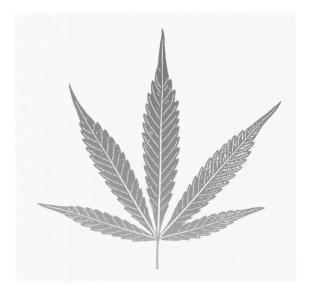

digestive tract and then the liver before it is absorbed into the blood. Where patients go wrong is not waiting long enough to judge effects. Sometimes they'll feel nothing after an hour or so and take another edible. Bad idea!

- There's another factor at play: Once the liver processes cannabis, it turns delta-9 THC into another compound, delta-11 THC, which is twice as strong and lasts twice as long as other methods of intake.
- The third reason is the result of prohibition: Because cannabis is still federally illegal, there is little consistency among edible products. In medical states, doses are clearly labeled, but even then, there are no standards. For example: a bar of chocolate may say "100 mg THC." It's up to you to know that if your optimum dose is 5 mg, you must divide that candy into 20 pieces. Again, knowing your dose and knowing how to read a label are key.

Add in increments of 2.5 mg, which is about the lowest quantity you'll find, and make sure to begin the process at night. This will help ensure a good night's sleep, and you'll wake up refreshed if you

mouth for quicker relief, and applied to skin for local conditions. Read labels carefully to see how many milligrams of cannabinoids a dropper contains. A good starting dose for CBD is 20-25 mg twice a day.

■ EDIBLES

Remember pot brownies? Besides that sickly, grassy taste, there was always one other big problem with these confections: You never knew what would happen. Take too little and nothing; too much and you're cowering in a corner for waaay too long.

Those days are over, thanks to dosed edibles. As medicine, they provide long-lasting relief–six to eight hours–to patients with pain or insomniacs in desperate need of a full night's sleep. Since very few edibles are pure CBD, the key to smart use is knowing how much to take.

Dosing edibles can be confusing to many patients, experienced or inexperienced. There are three reasons why:

- Effects take one to two hours to kick in, because anything you eat must first pass through the

Sample dosing schedule for edibles with recommended milligrams of THC							
	M	**T**	**W**	**TH**	**F**	**SA**	**SU**
AM	0	0	2.5	2.5	2.5	2.5	2.5
PM	2.5	2.5	2.5	2.5	5.0	5.0	5.0

NOTE This sample patient used medical edibles for long-lasting relief but supplemented them with inhalations whenever she felt breakthrough pain.

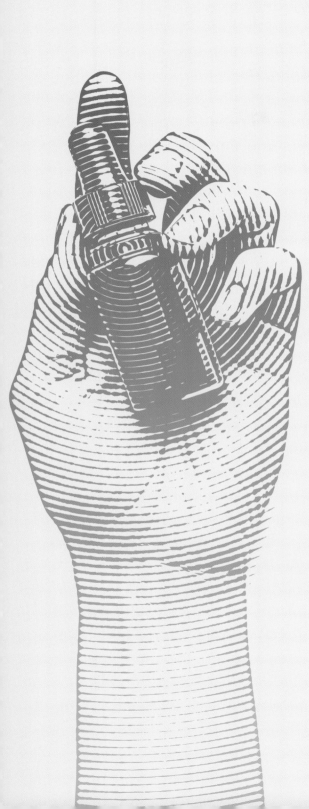

don't take too much. Here's a sample of a THC edible-dosing schedule used by a patient with pain and insomnia. It's a good place to begin.

■ TOPICALS

Topicals come as salves, sprays, lotions, unguents, pain patches...all of which are simple to use and have no psychoactivity.

Cannabis pain patches work differently and are excellent for more systemic issues. Just like other pain patches, they deliver active ingredients directly into the bloodstream through the skin. Pain patches are not a "spot treatment," so if you have back pain, it's not necessary to apply it to your back. Placing it on your upper arm will do the trick. Effects will be felt somewhere between 15 and 30 minutes and can last between eight and 10 hours.

Important: Pain patches come in various strengths and ratios of THC:CBD, but they also typically come in walloping doses of THC. Once you know your optimal dose, it makes sense to simply cut patches into smaller sizes.

■ WHAT IF YOU TAKE TOO MUCH?

You can't overdose and die from taking too much cannabis—that's the good news. However, you can overconsume THC, which may bring on lethargy, paranoia, distorted thoughts, and, in rare cases, vomiting. Seventeen percent of new users report experiencing some type of adverse reactions.

So, what do you do if you take too much? Other than staying calm, breathing deeply and relaxing, the best remedy is a spray bottle of CBD, which helps to cut the effects of THC. A few sprays of CBD under your tongue, swished around your mouth for five or 10 minutes, will reduce discomfort and restore you to a more balanced state.

–Joe Dolce

Joe Dolce is the author of Brave New Weed: Adventures into the Uncharted World of Cannabis *and the founder of medicalmannabismentor.com, an online education course.*

GIVING PHYSICIANS A NEW PRESCRIPTION

DOCTORS ARE FINALLY STARTING TO UNDERSTAND THE BENEFITS OF CBD.

After her fibromyalgia flared up, Kimmy Seegmiller asked her doctor about CBD oil to help control her pain. "I wanted something besides Lyrica, which had bad side effects for me," she explains. Her question was met with an unwelcome response.

"He basically said that marijuana doesn't work, and there was no proof," reveals Seegmiller. The Missouri native went on to research medical cannabis herself before purchasing a bottle of cannabidiol (CBD) oil online. (CBD oil is one of 104 chemical compounds known as cannabinoids found in the cannabis plant.) She noticed nearly immediate results with zero side effects.

"I have a lot less pain, and the aches in my joints are gone," she says. Not surprisingly, Seegmiller is

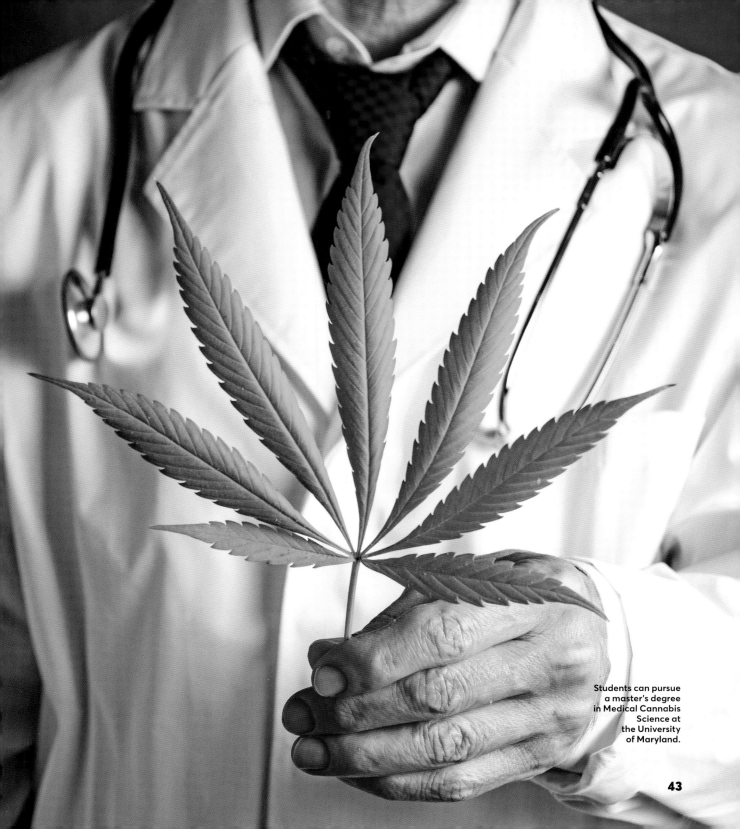

Students can pursue
a master's degree
in Medical Cannabis
Science at
the University
of Maryland.

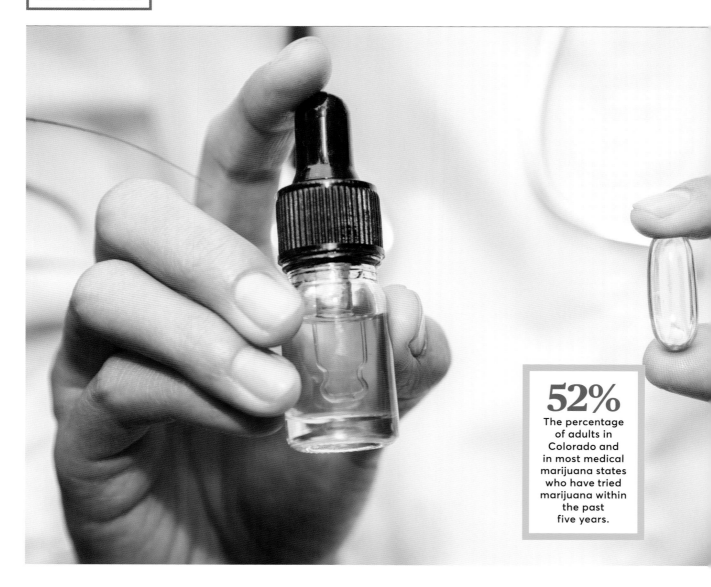

52%
The percentage
of adults in
Colorado and
in most medical
marijuana states
who have tried
marijuana within
the past
five years.

glad she took matters into her own hands but remains frustrated by the lack of knowledge on the subject by her regular doctor. "I felt like I was asking for something illegal or doing something wrong because I was trying to get better instead of being dependent on pharmaceutical companies."

■ GATHERING THE EVIDENCE

This disconnect between doctors and medical cannabis continues, even as medical marijuana becomes more socially acceptable. CBD-based products may, in fact, have an easier time getting both medical and social approval because, unlike

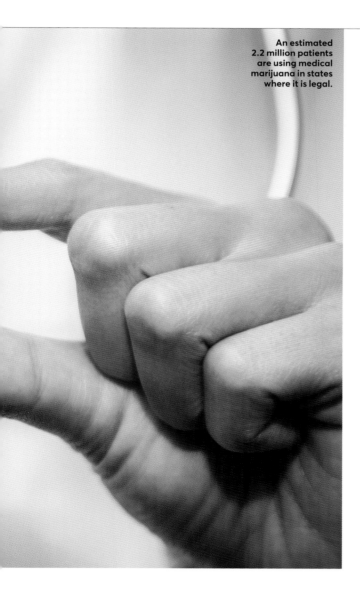

Science is catching on: There's strong evidence CBD can help as an anti-seizure medication. In June 2018, the FDA approved Epidiolex, the first cannabis-derived medicine for epilepsy that contains CBD. It's also commonly used to address insomnia, with studies showing CBD may help patients fall asleep faster and stay asleep.

One of the most popular uses, though, is to help treat various types of chronic pain. Scientists say CBD may work by activating or inhibiting other compounds in the body's endocannabinoid system, which helps to regulate functions such as sleep, immune-system responses and pain. Research has shown that CBD may help reduce pain perception while curbing inflammation in the brain and nervous system. A 2017 report from the National Academies of Sciences, Engineering and Medicine found that adults with chronic pain treated with CBD were more likely to experience a significant reduction in symptoms.

▪ CONTINUING CANNABIS EDUCATION

Some health professionals are working to educate clinicians about the potential health benefits of CBD and the ins and outs of medical marijuana. "We're putting together continuing education for doctors, to give them more information about the pros, the cons and the evidence that we have," says Michelle H. Cameron, MD, PT, MCR, at the Department of Neurology of Oregon Health & Science University.

Ira Price, MD, assistant clinical professor in the Division of Emergency Medicine through the Department of Internal Medicine at Canada's McMaster University, has been working on this information gap. He started the Association of Cannabis Specialists (ACS), an international group aimed at educating cannabis specialists and referring clinicians.

"One of the most fascinating aspects of the medical cannabis industry is it was not a pharmacy nor a doctor leading the way for change—it was the patient," he says. "As far as I know, there are no major medical schools addressing either the science of the endocannabinoid system or the therapeutic use of cannabis. This has to—and will—change, but it'll take time."

marijuana, they come primarily from the hemp plant and don't contain any of the "high"-inducing chemical THC (tetrahydrocannabinol). It's also become readily available in most of the U.S., with all 50 states passing laws that legalize CBD with varying degrees of restriction.

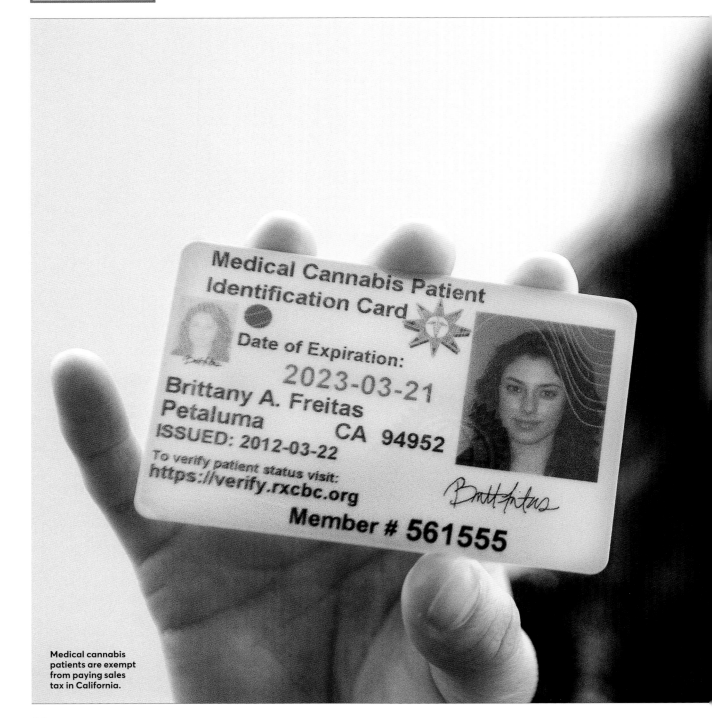

Medical cannabis patients are exempt from paying sales tax in California.

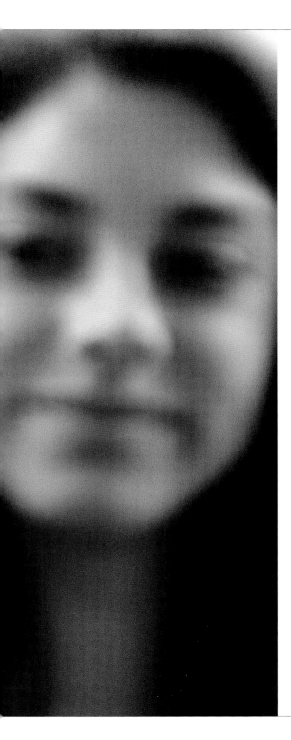

GETTING CARDED

EVERYTHING YOU ALWAYS NEEDED TO KNOW ABOUT GETTING YOUR FIRST MEDICAL-MARIJUANA CARD—BUT WERE AFRAID TO ASK.

Medical marijuana is now legal in 33 states and Washington D.C., but in order to obtain cannabis for your health, you'll need a medical card granting you access. So how do you go about obtaining one? We spoke with an expert, Rob Tankson, founder and CEO of prestodoctor.com, in order to learn more. Tankson's organization provides online cannabis evaluations from doctors, as well as treatment plans for patients in California, Nevada and New York.

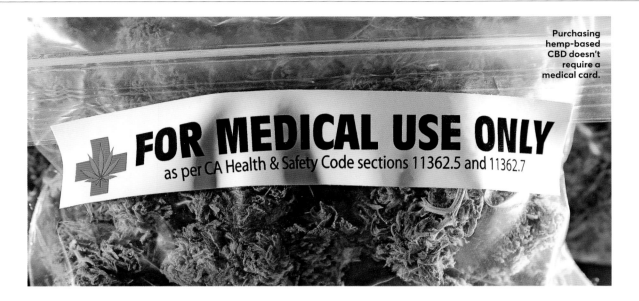

Purchasing hemp-based CBD doesn't require a medical card.

FOR MEDICAL USE ONLY
as per CA Health & Safety Code sections 11362.5 and 11362.7

How do you go about getting a medical marijuana card?

You first need to be evaluated by a physician. Some people go to their primary doctor, but most see a doctor who specializes in medical-cannabis evaluations because a dispensary must verify the recommendation—which can take longer with a typical doctor than with a specialist who already has an automated system in place. An online evaluation is easiest, but you can Google for medical marijuana evaluations near you, or search leafly.com's doctor locator.

What does it cost and how long will it last?

It varies. Some evaluations are as low as $40, while others cost up to $150. We charge $70 in California and $50 for returning patients.

In California, the doctor gives you the necessary paperwork to enter a dispensary, but in most every other state, the state issues you a card or paperwork, usually in a matter of minutes or hours. Most states do charge a registration fee, from $1 in Washington State to $200 in Oregon. A card is typically good for one year in most states.

What are qualifying conditions?

In some states, you have to have a terminal illness, but in many states, chronic pain or PTSD will qualify you; even anxiety qualifies in California.

Does insurance cover any of it?

Not currently.

How do I go about finding a dispensary?

Just go online and Google for medical marijuana dispensaries in your state. They're even rated, just like most other types of businesses that you search.

How do you know what strain to use, and how much?

Almost 50 percent of the patients we see are new to cannabis, and it can be daunting—there areso many questions. We give every patient a personalized treatment plan that says, "You have this condition; this is what the doctor recommends, and you should consume it this way [by vaping, as edibles or in tinctures]. You should do it this often and at this time of day." We typically recommend "microdosing" initially, 2.5 to 5 mg, to see how it affects you, then waiting half a day. Since, legally, doctors have to give a recommendation and not a prescription, it's as close as we can get to providing a prescription.

Do you need to get a medical marijuana card in the seven states where cannabis is now fully legal?

Yes. There are a couple reasons of you'd want to get a card. The best one: If you spend more than $100 a month, you'll save money with a tax break of at least 7.5 percent—even higher in some counties in California.

Can you buy medical marijuana at recreational dispensaries in states where pot is legal?

It varies. In Colorado, there are dispensaries just for medical and just for recreational, but in California and Nevada, most of the dispensaries are one-stop shops.

Many states allow you to grow your own if you have a card—which is how much marijuana, generally?

It differs by state and even by county. In California, some counties allow growing; some don't. Some states allow patients to grow plants—the number is typically anywhere from six to 12—but only some of those can be mature plants.

And how much can you possess?

It's all over the map, so to speak. Most states limit you to some amount of dried marijuana, but some are more generous with the amount than others—so it's important to check your state's laws.

What does a dried ounce typically cost in a dispensary?

It's a lot like wine: The higher the quality, the higher the cost. But you expect to pay about $30 to $35 for average quality. For higher-quality buds, the price can go up to $400 an ounce.

Concentrates like waxes and oils for vaping are $20 to $60 a gram. Edibles come in all kinds of foods now—pizza, burritos, ice cream, you name it—and

In some states, you must have a terminal illness (to get a medical card); but in many states, chronic pain or PTSD will qualify you."

ROB TANKSON,
CEO OF PRESTODOCTOR.COM

cost about $3 to $5 per dose, but you don't need as much, and they last longer. Liquid concentrates or tinctures, which you can put in foods or beverages, cost between $20 and $40 for a 1-oz bottle.

Last question: are there any other pitfalls to consider with medical cannabis?

Your permit to carry a concealed firearm might be in jeopardy, but that varies from state to state. In Nevada, your concealed-carry permit will be revoked if you're listed on the state medical-marijuana registry, but that's not the case in New York, California or Oregon.

Typically, state law trumps federal law, but until the federal government reclassifies cannabis, there will always be some conflict. Also, many nationwide or global companies, like airlines, may have policies that prohibit marijuana use and will test for it.

PEACE STRAINS

THERE ARE MANY TYPES OF MARIJUANA THAT COULD POTENTIALLY SOOTHE AND HEAL. HERE'S A BREAKDOWN OF SOME OF THE MOST POPULAR.

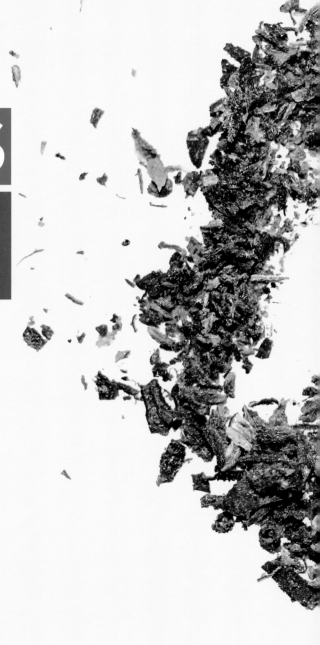

When you get right down to it, marijuana is kind of like the Meryl Streep of the plant world. Both are exceedingly popular. Both are very good at what they do. And just when you think you've got them typecast in a role, they show up as something that's new and completely different.

In Ms. Streep's case, these traits bring lots of Oscars. In the case of cannabis, they can bring peace and comfort to those suffering from a variety of illnesses. For the past several decades, a large percentage of Americans have marginalized marijuana

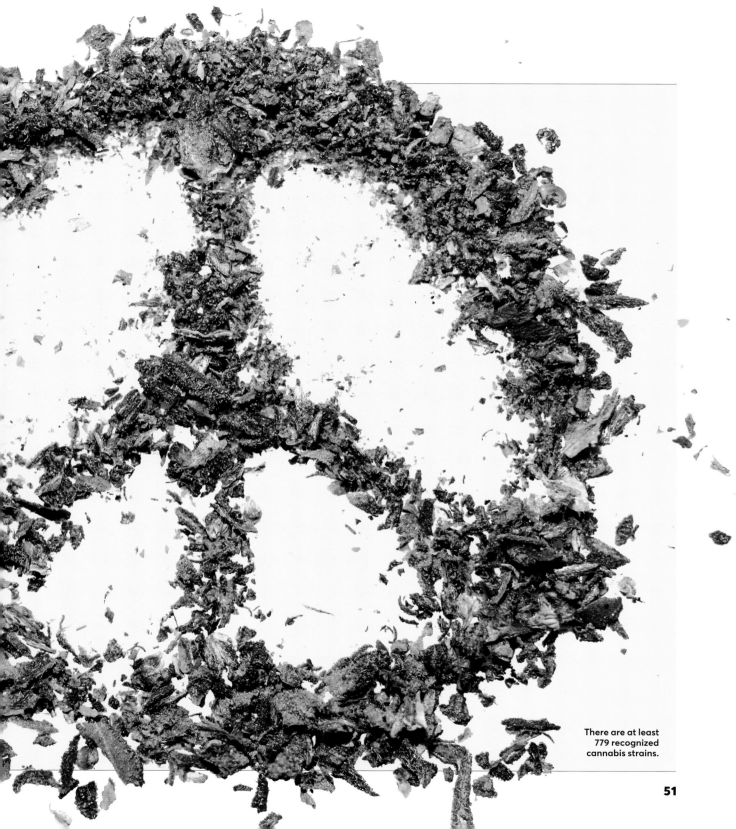

There are at least
779 recognized
cannabis strains.

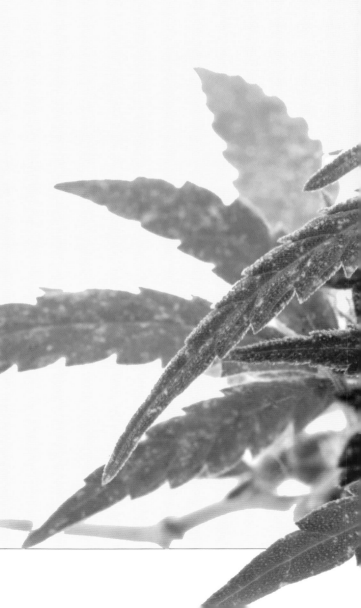

as that thing college roommates and famous musicians use to escape reality for a while. However, as state after state adopts medical-marijuana programs, the plant has now morphed into something that may help with everything from depression to epilepsy to cancer.

The best-known cannabis strain cultivated for medicinal use is probably Charlotte's Web. It is named after Charlotte Figi, a young girl with a severe form of epilepsy who was the first patient treated with oil produced from this strain. Raised for its high CBD content and extremely low levels of THC (the chemical in cannabis that produces the infamous high), Charlotte's Web had its profile raised after Dr. Sanjay Gupta followed the young patient's progress for a CNN report.

■ GROWING WEED LIKE WINE

With increasing interest in medicinal use, more American growers are developing cannabis strains that are cannabinoid-rich. There's very little documented scientific data to go on, so they have been forced to rely on holistic techniques to refine their strains. Similar to vintage wines, strains are often developed not only for effect but also for combinations of terpenes (hydrocarbons found in the essential oils of many plants) that add flavor and scent. Terpenes and other plant compounds also enhance the effect of the cannabinoids that may produce the desired medical effects. For reputable cannabis growers, cultivation without the use of pesticides is a priority, to protect patients who may already be immune-compromised.

Fanciful strain names are limited only by the grower's imagination. Cannabis plants are typically referred to as feminine, since the female plants produce flowers that can then be smoked or distilled into oil. Those oils are then added to tinctures, topical applications or edibles or loaded into oil cartridges for patients who vape. We asked several experts to suggest the most effective medical strains available.

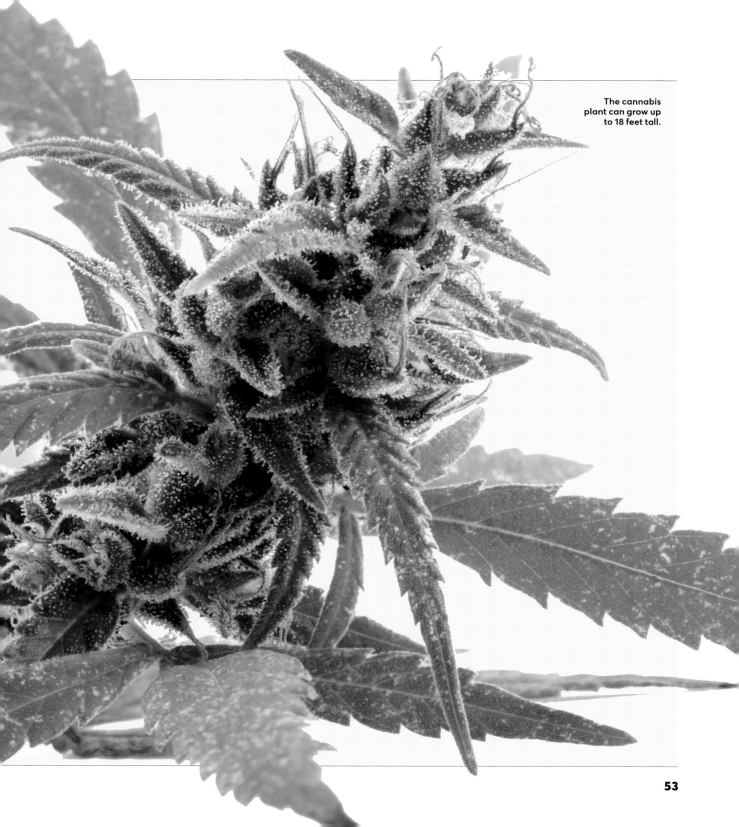

The cannabis plant can grow up to 18 feet tall.

EVALUATING EFFECTIVE MEDICAL MARIJUANA STRAINS

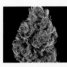

ACDC

"Also commonly called Charlotte's Web, this classic CBD-dominant variety rose to notoriety due to its reported effectiveness in controlling seizures associated with epilepsy. While ACDC can be a difficult plant to cultivate, its flower is consistently pleasant, with notes of sweet grass and light citrus." —Walker

BLUE DRAGON DESERT FROST

"It's a flower born of a single coveted miracle seed that was gifted to us by a patient who swore that it was the best for her anxiety and pain and wanted a steady supply. We got lucky that it was female and an amazing rare strain. She tests at around 15–18 percent CBD and 1 percent THC, so one might not initially believe her strong CBD dominance by smell alone. Trichomes-laden purple buds bring a subtle euphoria and relief." —Rivero

CHEM 4

"A high-THC strain, this has had great success treating pain. Chem 4 is also high in the plant compound beta-myrcene. This combination tends to help patients with a lot of pain. Chem 4 tests for THC in the high 20 percent range and packs a punch with its terpene profile. Most use it at night for pain control before bed." —Peters

CORAZON

"Rich in CBD, Corazon has a way of earning a soft spot in your heart. We have been donating this particular strain to a young patient with severe epilepsy, and it seems to be the only one that works for him. He has gone from many seizures every day to nearly zero, allowing him to ride his bike again and enjoy life. With a 20:1 ratio of CBD to THC, it's no wonder this strain works wonders; but there is definitely a bit of magic involved as well." —Rivero

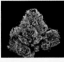

DOSIDO

"This strain packs a powerful psychoactive punch, with an immediate calming body stone coupled with a heavy mental space that is deeply relaxing and offers instant pain relief to many. One of our most beautiful and trichomes-caked cultivars, this one boasts a rare non-myrcene-dominant terpene profile with nerolidol and limonene." —Rivero

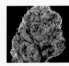

LEMMIWINKS

"With its potent, sweet grape-flavored buds, Lemmiwinks is one of our top strains for relaxation and sleep. One of my personal go-tos to help with muscle spasms and pain I have due to nerve issues. The calming effect is perfect after a hard day at work; it's a great nighttime smoke." —Sloat

LSD

"LSD (not to be confused with the drug best known for its psychological effects) is a high-THC strain that has had success stopping seizures when converted to RSO (Rick Simpson Oil). To date, we have not been able to nail down what part of the profile is so unique, but it seems to work. The genotype we have is exceptionally difficult to grow, but in the end, we keep her around specifically for her medicinal purposes." —Peters

MAUI BUBBLE GIFT

"This has a 2:1 ratio, CBD to THC. MBG is one of our most popular medicinal strains. It's a rare variety that's easy to have issues with; if treated well, it grows strong. We have many patients who have treated a host of issues with great success. Her cannabinoid and terpene profile seems to treat people very well. Patients have used it for Parkinson's disease, cerebral palsy and cancer." —Peters

PINEAPPLE JAGER

"We bred this variety by combining a southern Oregon favorite strain called Jager (aka Purple Hindu Kush) with Pineapple Tsu. The result is a 3:1 CBD-to-THC plant, packed with a diverse range of terpenes. The high terpene content rounds out the cannabinoids for a potent yet comfortable array of effects. A considerable nose stands out in this variety, with notes of tropical fruit and 'fuel' coming through the strongest." —Walker

PLATINUM TIGER COOKIES

"A high-THC/sativa hybrid for relaxation, both physical and mental. The sativa influences of this strain can cause the giggles, which makes it perfect for social settings or enjoying a private moment. The touch of indica takes away any edge or paranoia-inducing aspects. Has a unique cheesy, lemony funk flavor." —Sloat

RINGO'S GIFT

"It's a legendary CBD powerhouse named after the late Lawrence Ringo, a pioneer in CBD-rich cannabis breeding and development. (A California native, he started growing cannabis at age 15 for back pain.) Ringo's Gift has been noted for its alleged association with clear-headed pain relief. This variety produces a dense flower with a peppery nose." —Walker

SISTER WIFE

"This has a 20:1 ratio, CBD to THC. It smells like blueberries and has a unique pinecone look. The high amount of CBD is great for inflammation and pain disorders, while the low THC (0.05 percent or less) helps relax the muscles and mind. It's also particularly good for menstrual cramps." —Sloat

SNOOP'S DREAM

"This is good for the 'introduction to cannabis' smoker, who wants to put a toe in the water. Cannabis is not the answer for everyone, but this is a great strain to start with—especially for those who are wary of the anxiety or paranoia sometimes associated with cannabis use. A cross of Master Kush and Blue Dream, the terpene profile is good for anxiety, PTSD or panic attacks." —Peters

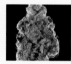

STRAWBERRY SATORI

"This variety shows high levels of linalool, a terpene that is commonly found in lavender. Early evidence suggests it may be effective against anxiety and stress, particularly in PTSD. Traditionally a THC-dominant variety, we're working to breed a CBD-rich variety that maintains the linalool profile. Characterized by its large flower structure, Strawberry Satori has a savory fruit nose, backed by notes of leather." —Walker

THE EXPERTS Dan Sloat Founder of the Colorado farm Alpinstash **Mason Walker** CEO of Oregon's East Fork Cultivars **Jesse Peters** Owner of the Oregon-based Eco Firma Farms **Laura Day Rivero** Operations Manager for Yerba Buena Farms, in Oregon

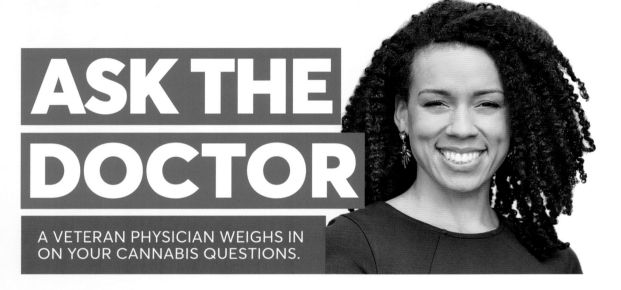

Dr. Rachel Knox operates American Cannabinoid Clinics along with her mom, dad and sister. See their story on page 176.

ASK THE DOCTOR

A VETERAN PHYSICIAN WEIGHS IN ON YOUR CANNABIS QUESTIONS.

The more we learn about the healing powers of cannabis, the more we realize we don't really know. That's why we ran some common questions about cannabis use by Rachel Knox, MD. Dr. Knox works with American Cannabinoid Clinics, which offers patient-centered, integrative cannabinoid care to patients looking for a personalized approach to addressing their health and healing.

Are doctors allowed to prescribe cannabis to patients they feel could benefit from it?

Doctors in the U.S. are not allowed to "prescribe" cannabis, as it is unlawful for physicians to prescribe Schedule 1 drugs in this country. But not only this, there is no current mechanism by which a physician would prescribe a Schedule 1 drug, as there are no legal distribution centers who could process those prescriptions. In the case of cannabis distribution in legal medical cannabis states, dispensaries do not operate like pharmacies, where a physician "prescription" can be filled according to the clinical directions written therein.

As it currently stands, medical-cannabis states will grant permission and protections through legislation to specified provider types to evaluate patients to determine eligibility or to authorize permission for cannabis use. An authorization for use simply grants a patient access to the legal market but does not function as a prescription that outlines product and dosing directions.

Physicians in most medical-cannabis states are allowed to consult with their patients, and discuss what the scientific literature has revealed or clinical relevance. In this way, patients can receive some direction on how to use their cannabis products beyond the authorization.

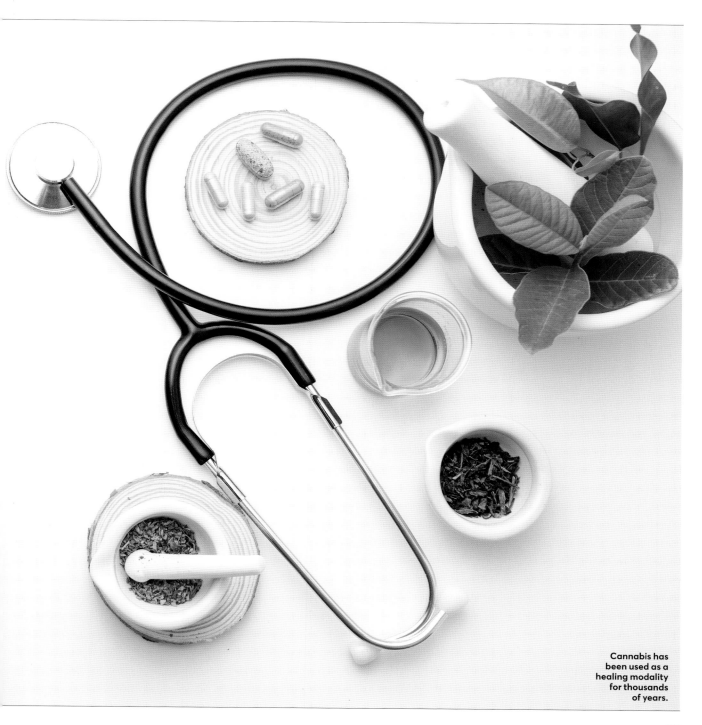

Cannabis has been used as a healing modality for thousands of years.

How do I know how much cannabis would be too much for me? Is there any way to know before I try it?

There are currently no approved tests to determine how a person may react to any given cannabis product. That being said, the unwanted side effects from cannabis–e.g., dry mouth, red eyes, racing heart, increased anxiety, paranoia, transient elevation in blood pressure, etc.–are attributed to the intoxicating and euphoric effects of the phytocannabinoid, THC [delta-9-tetrahydrocannabinol]. A person may know that they have had "too much" if they experience these symptoms to a degree that is unwanted or uncomfortable for them. "Too much" THC is a subjective experience.

And not everyone experiences one or more of these side effects. But to avoid them, patient-consumers–what I like to call the average cannabis consumer–should limit the amount of THC internally consumed [inhaled, ingested, or inoculated in some other internal manner through mucosal membranes, such as in the mouth or anus/vagina].

A common mantra throughout the industry with regards to consumption is to "start low and go slow." This means a person should start with a small amount of THC, increasing over time to determine the "minimally effective dose," or the lowest concentration of THC a person wants to tolerate while achieving the desired effects.

I love working out and doing a lot of running. How does using cannabis affect my ability to get a good workout?

The long answer to this question is highly nuanced and scientific. The short answer is that a person needs to be aware of the effects that cannabis use has on them individually. Listening to the body–honing in on how it responds positively or negatively to foods, supplements, water and even cannabis (and the various methods of cannabis consumption) with respect to exercise–is the best way to determine how cannabis affects one's ability to achieve a good workout.

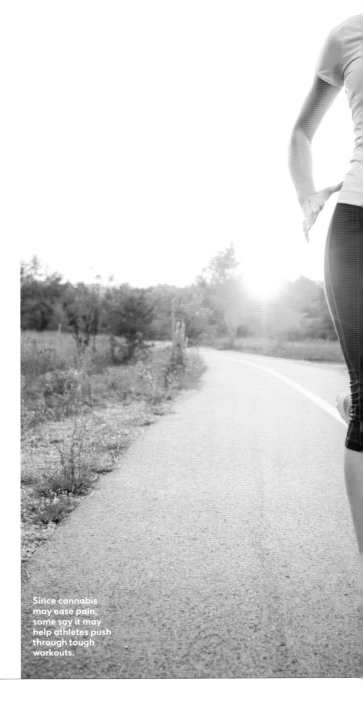

Since cannabis may ease pain, some say it may help athletes push through tough workouts.

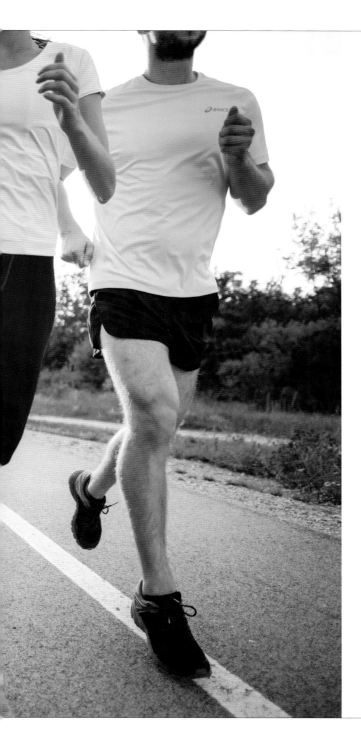

For example, if smoking cannabis before your workout reduces your lung capacity (the amount of air filling the lungs) during intense intervals, the conclusion may be that smoking cannabis is a hindrance to your workout. Conversely, as THC is a bronchodilator, if smoking cannabis before your workout improves your lung capacity, the conclusion may be that smoking cannabis is a benefit to your workout. As with any experience with cannabis, how its use might affect exercise is a highly individualized one.

I'd heard that if I wanted to lose weight, smoking weed would be helpful. Is that true? Does cannabis help reduce appetite?

A side effect of THC is increased appetite, while several studies suggest that the cannabinoids CBD and THCV can suppress it. That being said, it is what a person eats or doesn't that has the most impact on weight gain and weight loss. For starters, dairy,

IS IT TRUE THAT CANNABIS CAN HURT MY SEX LIFE?

It is true that cannabis can affect libido or physical function, but that occurs on a case-by-case basis and often in the setting of misuse—that is, overuse or abuse— and can typically be mitigated through adjusting consumption practices.

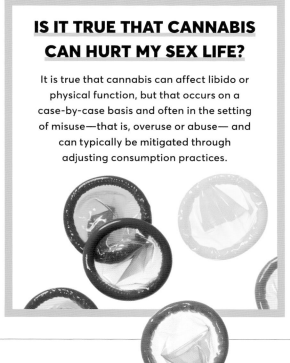

grain, vegetable oils and sugar are the primary food groups responsible for weight gain, for myriad reasons. Two of those reasons are that these food groups cause inflammation and insulin imbalance in the body. Cannabis and cannabinoids can help combat inflammation, but if you're interested in losing weight, cut these foods out of your diet.

We hear all about how cannabis can help with serious illnesses like epilepsy, Parkinson's disease and dementia. But are there any benefits cannabis provides for more common ailments, like colds and flu?
Colds and flu are caused by viruses. Some cannabinoids have antiseptic properties, meaning that they have been observed to prevent the growth of disease-causing microorganisms like bacteria and viruses at varying concentrations, but what's more interesting is the role cannabinoids can play in balancing the immune system.

A strong immune system is one's leading line of defense in fighting colds and flu. Many patient-consumers use cannabinoids preventively through regular use to maintain a healthy immune system and, in this way, indirectly prevent catching a cold or coming down with the flu. A person could also elect to use cannabis or cannabinoid products during a cold or flu for symptomatic relief or even immune support, but no research has validated the use of cannabis in the setting of acute illness to treat colds and flu. The same would

IS THERE ANY AGE THAT'S CONSIDERED TOO OLD TO USE CANNABIS, EITHER FOR FUN OR MEDICALLY?

The fastest-growing demographic of cannabis users in the U.S. is adults aged 55 and older. My guess is that most are turning to cannabis to address a medical or health-related need, but this isn't to say that an elderly patient-consumer cannot also enjoy their cannabis consumption. Caution should be taken, however, for patient-consumers who are on multiple medications, have preexisting cognitive conditions or other physical limitations. There do exist drug-drug interactions with cannabis, and the effects of "too much" THC can potentially lead to unwanted cognitive changes or imbalance, for example. This can be mitigated through proper counsel and by choosing the right products and chemical profiles, routes of administration and time of use.

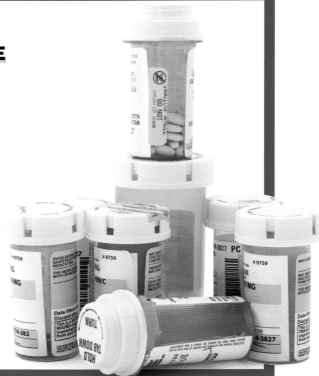

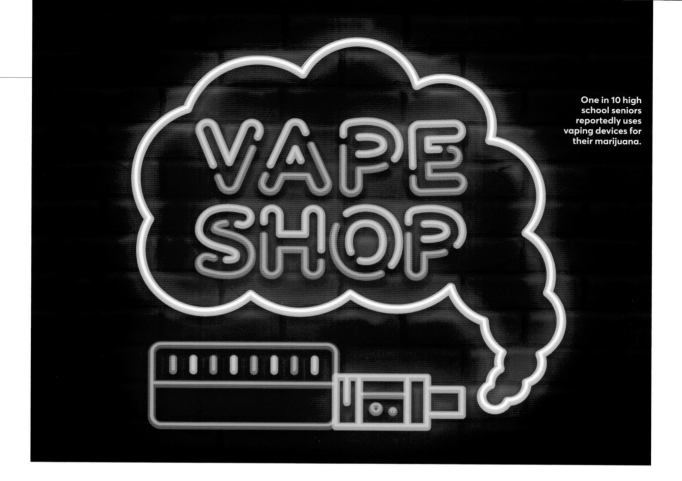

One in 10 high school seniors reportedly uses vaping devices for their marijuana.

likely be true of other common ailments that correlate with the health of one's immune state.

Is smoking cannabis worse for me than smoking cigarettes?

Emphatically, no! In fact, research led by Dr. Donald Tashkin at UCLA showed that cannabis does not increase risk for serious lung diseases such as lung cancer, emphysema and respiratory infection compared to nonsmokers—even despite evidence that cannabis smoke does contain some nasty carcinogens and combustion by-products. Theories for this finding are based on the anticancer effects of the cannabis plant's phytocannabinoids.

It should be noted though that Dr. Tashkin's research did identify some negative outcomes for long-term cannabis smokers. Specifically, long-time cannabis smokers did have more chronic bronchitis than nonsmokers—that is, they experienced irritated airways, sore throat, wheezing and cough. But these ill effects are reversible and non-life-threatening. Cannabis smokers experiencing these side effects should decrease or eliminate smoking of cannabis and try gentler administration methods, such as vaporization, tinctures or edibles.

Is vaping better for me than smoking cannabis?

The jury is still out on this one: We need to collect and analyze empirical and scientific data to properly assess the long-term health effects associated with the use of e-cigarettes and other vaping products on the market.

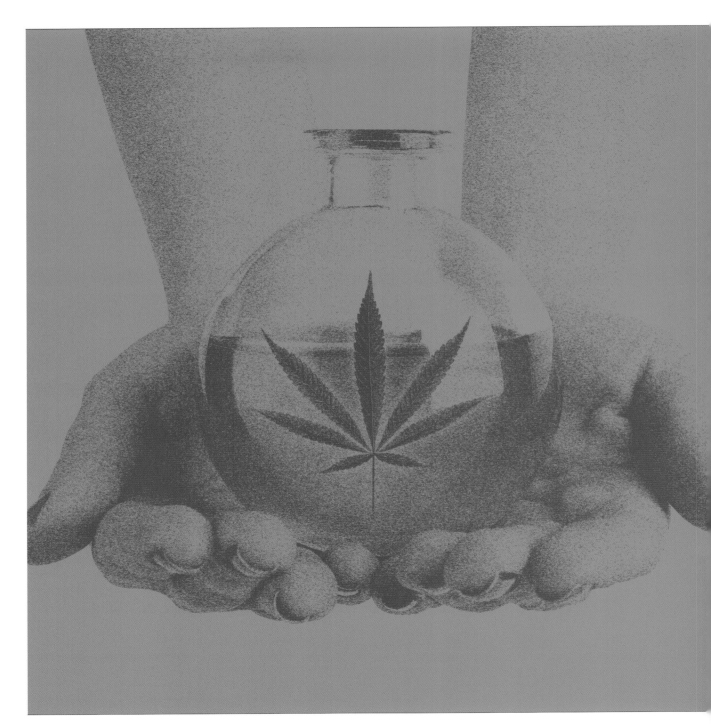

PART 2

HEALING POWER

A-Z CANNABIS GUIDE TO HEALING

FROM ALZHEIMER'S TO ZOSTER, THIS COMPREHENSIVE LIST LOOKS AT A VARIETY OF AILMENTS AND WHAT, IF ANY, RELIEF CANNABIS CAN HELP PROVIDE.

No matter where we're from, who we voted for or whether we're more of a dog or a cat person, there are two things pretty much all of us have in common. First, at some point in our lives, we're going to get sick. And second, we've recently read about, or discussed with someone, the medicinal potential of marijuana. Cannabis has started to seem like a miracle drug, the cure for whatever ails us. Americans have come to believe so much in the reported healing powers of this plant that one poll found that more than 90 percent of adults want medical marijuana legalized on the federal level.

Still, solid research is not easy to come by. It can be difficult to separate fact from fiction when it comes to determining what marijuana can help with. So, we spoke to cannabis experts Emma Chasen, Mary Brown, Dr. Bonni Goldstein and Dr. Mary Clifton to get their thoughts on the conditions for which this plant might provide relief.

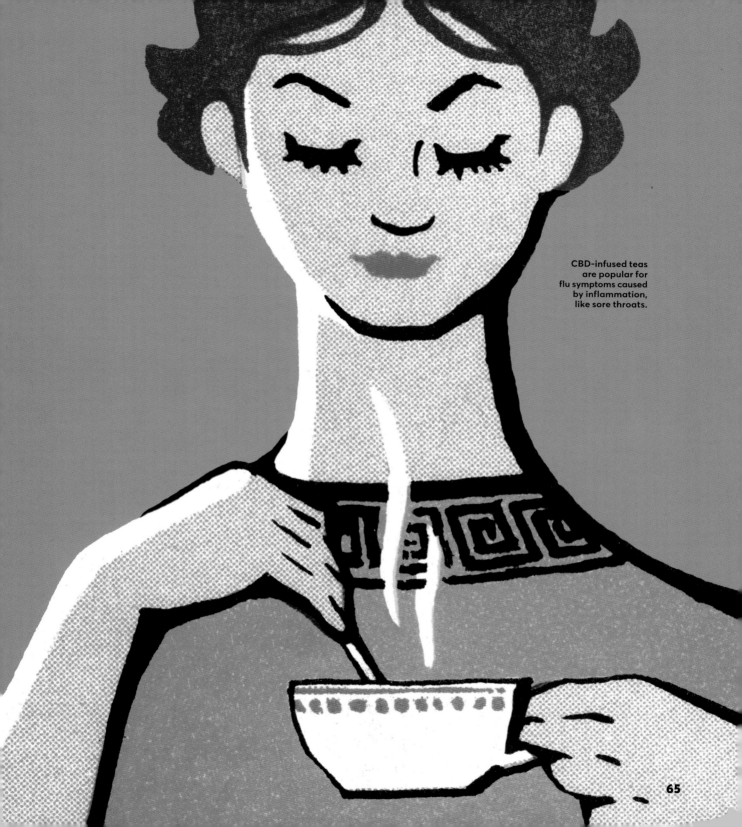

CBD-infused teas are popular for flu symptoms caused by inflammation, like sore throats.

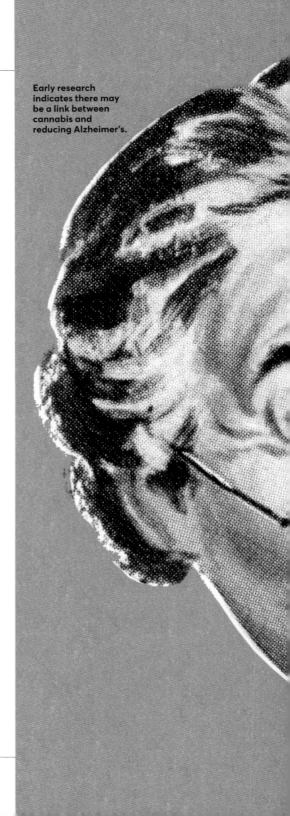

Early research indicates there may be a link between cannabis and reducing Alzheimer's.

Cannabis Experts

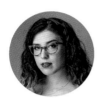

EMMA CHASEN
A graduate of Brown University with a degree in medicinal plant research, Chasen has worked as general manager and director of education for the popular Portland, Oregon, dispensary Farma. She now operates Eminent Consulting, which offers cannabis education for those in the industry as well as for medical and recreational users.

MARY BROWN
Brown works as the executive director and lead consultant for the Seattle-based SMJ Consulting at the AIMS Institute, which offers medical patients education services and individualized wellness programs that are centered on cannabinoid therapy.

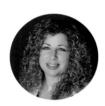

DR. BONNI GOLDSTEIN
The former chief resident at Children's Hospital Los Angeles, she is now the director of the California-based Canna-Centers, a wellness organization that educates patients on the use of cannabis for serious and chronic conditions. Goldstein is also the author of the book *Cannabis Revealed.*

DR. MARY CLIFTON
CBD and cannabis expert Clifton is an internal medicine doctor with more than 20 years of experience. She is now a leading voice in telemedicine, and offers consultations through her website, cbdandcannabisinfo.com. Clifton is also the author of *The Grass Is Greener: Medical Marijuana, THC & CBD Oil: Reversing Chronic Pain, Inflammation and Disease.*

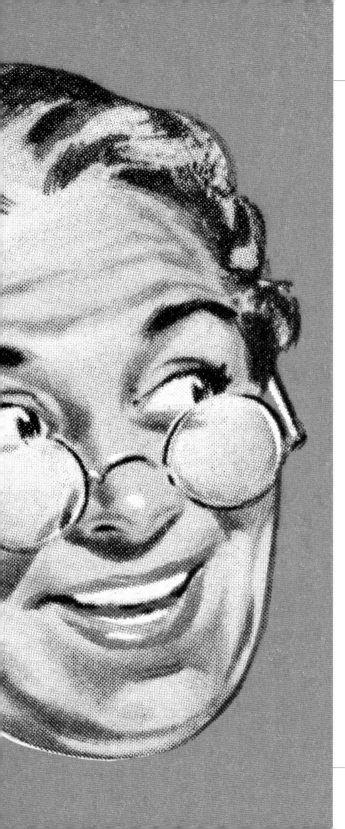

◄ Alzheimer's Disease

There have been preclinical trials—using mice—that Goldstein says are very encouraging when it comes to treating this illness with cannabis, adding that "what's unknown is what dose might stabilize or reverse the disease." Says Brown, "Cannabinoids may be helpful in stopping the buildup of plaque in the brain that contributes to Alzheimer's. CBD, CBG and microdosing THC are effective cannabinoid therapies."

Anorexia

According to Chasen, "THC has been linked to appetite stimulation and may be able to help anorexic patients eat." However, because anorexia is a psychological disorder, Brown emphasizes that it is also important to consult with a doctor about treatment. Goldstein adds that anorexia nervosa patients have seen some success with a combination of CBD and THC, because they can "help with those perseverating thoughts" associated with the illness.

Anxiety

CBD, as well as the cannabinoid CBG, have shown potential in helping to treat anxiety, explains Brown. But it's a tricky situation. On the one hand, Clifton says there has been at least one significant study that indicated some cannabis could improve the symptoms of anxiety. On the other, she notes that "you can sometimes aggravate [your anxiety] with a high-THC product or create a little paranoia."

B

Back Pain

The experts all agree that when it comes to easing chronic pain, CBD in particular can be very effective. And with the "entourage effect" that comes from throwing in other cannabinoids, "it could probably do even better," says Clifton. There's also the analgesic (muscle relaxing) properties of cannabis that Brown says can bring relief. Chasen notes that the use of topical medicines is best, because they can be applied right to the point of pain.

C

Common Cold

As great as it would be to finally have a cure for the common cold, we'll have to wait a bit longer because, says Clifton, there's been no significant research into whether cannabis can help. However, as with other herbal treatments, she does say that "there is definitely immunity modulation that goes on [with cannabis] that probably helps reduce the intensity of the symptoms if you're taking it before you get sick."

Crohn's Disease

Thanks to the multitude of CB2 receptors in the lower abdominal organs, according to Brown, cannabinoids CBD and CBG could help ease the pain of Crohn's, especially when taken orally. Goldstein suggests using some degree of THC as well. Explains Chasen, "So many cannabis compounds can help calm the smooth muscle of the digestive system and help Crohn's patients more effectively manage their disease."

D

Depression ▶

"You'll probably see some benefit with THC and CBD, although there's less data on this than there is for anxiety," explains Clifton. They may work because the compounds within cannabis, adds Chasen, interact with our serotonin and dopamine systems, which modulate our mood. "CBD is a great low-risk option, especially when coupled with terpenes such as limonene and b-caryophyllene," she says. "THC may also be helpful. However, it can also heighten depressive symptoms if used in too high a concentration. Therefore, keep it low and go for something CBD-dominant."

Diabetes

While there's no concrete proof cannabis can cure this illness in humans, Goldstein says there has been a preclinical trial that looked into stopping type 1 diabetes with lab mice. "They found that if they started CBD very early after mice developed diabetes, they could reverse it," she explains. What cannabis can do for people, though, is help ease the pain of diabetes' side effects, such as retinal damage, diabetic neuropathy and nerve pain. In addition, she adds that it can have a positive effect on balancing the body's sugars, but it's also critical to eat better and exercise more, rather than just relying on cannabis alone.

Cannabis Health Tip

Inhaling medical marijuana will get it working quicker in your system. Ingesting it will take longer to work, but the effects also last longer.

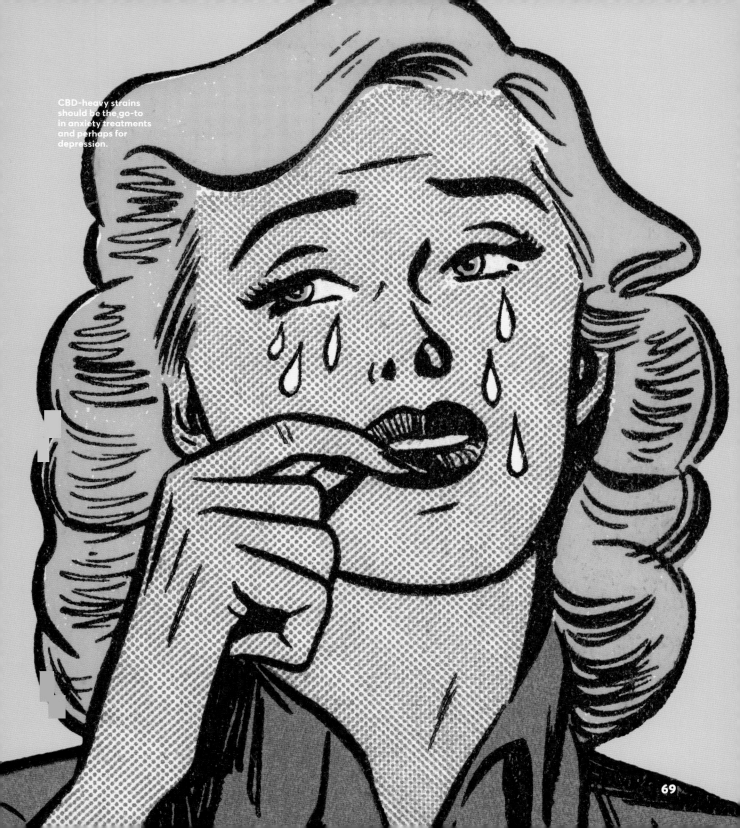

CBD-heavy strains should be the go-to in anxiety treatments and perhaps for depression.

E

Epilepsy

This is one condition that has been extensively studied, to the point where there's even an FDA-approved, cannabis-derived drug to help with seizures: Epidiolex. "High-CBD strains have been reported to greatly reduce seizure frequency, and THC has been included in reports as having potential for rescue during seizures," says Brown. While Clifton is encouraged by studies she's seen supporting this conclusion, she also cautions that the dosage required is "in the hundreds of milligrams."

F

Fibromyalgia

The anti-inflammatory and pain-mediation properties of cannabis make it a strong option for fibromyalgia sufferers. Brown cites a study of 390 participants with the illness where 62 percent reported cannabis as "very effective" in treating their symptoms and 33 percent reported that it helped "a little." As for what to take, she says that "the ratio of CBD to THC that benefits patients is based on individual preference."

Flu

As with a cold, cannabis can potentially help with "immune system response modulation"—meaning for it to do any good, you need to use it to help your body fight off the virus that can give you the flu. "There's no hard evidence that shows using cannabis while ill will make you get well quicker or block the severity of the illness," says Goldstein, adding that it can help flu sufferers sleep, lose some of their achiness and get their appetite back.

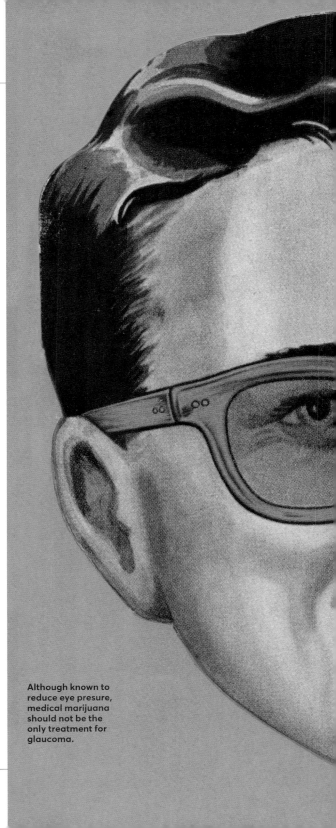

Although known to reduce eye presure, medical marijuana should not be the only treatment for glaucoma.

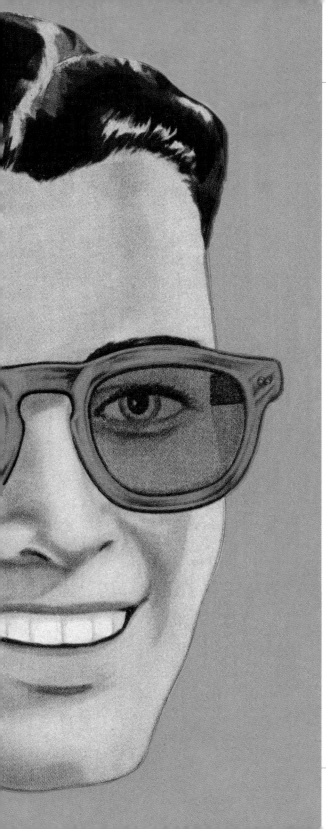

G

◀ Glaucoma

We've long known smoking cannabis can ease eye pressure and help glaucoma sufferers. "Through its analgesic and anti-inflammatory properties, cannabis can be used as a pain reliever and may reduce swelling of the optic nerve," says Brown. However, Goldstein cautions that "despite the fact that it's on every state [medical program] list of what can be approved for glaucoma, cannabis isn't mono therapy." Instead, it should be seen as "an adjunct" to other treatments recommended by your doctor.

H

Hepatitis

Because this condition results from having an inflamed liver, Clifton believes that cannabis can "have a proactive effect" if taken in low doses.

I

Insomnia

"Cannabis can act as an effective support for insomnia patients," says Brown. "CBN is a complementary cannabinoid to THC and CBD for enhancing the sleep-inducing effects." Chasen enthusiastically concurs. "THC and CBD can both help regulate sleep-cycling, though THC may keep you out of REM sleep," she explains. "Therefore, opt for a higher concentration of CBD compared to THC. Plus, terpenes like linalool can really help get you to sleep–and help you stay asleep!"

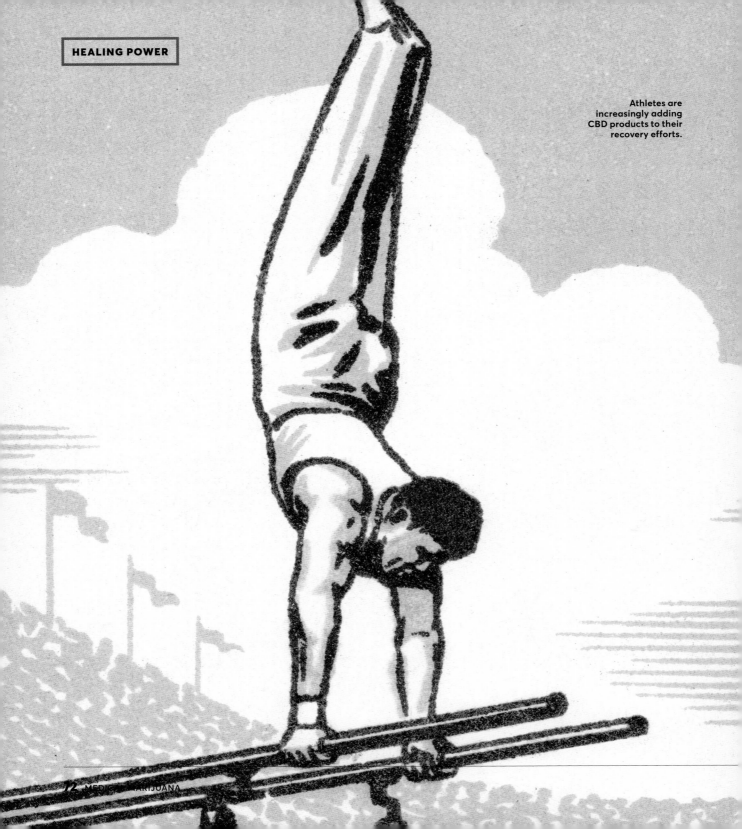

Athletes are increasingly adding CBD products to their recovery efforts.

Jock Itch

This isn't a job for cannabis or CBD directly, according to Clifton. However, using a compound such as pinene or limonene that's included in a topical, such as a salve or lotion, can have an antibacterial effect, which may not only ease jock itch but also outbreaks of things like toe fungus.

Kidney Disease

Cannabinoids like THC and CBD are able to pass through the kidney's filtration system but stop to interact with the cannabinoid receptors that regulate kidney function. THC also appears to help manage chronic pain among patients with chronic kidney disease, according to a study published in the *Canadian Journal of Kidney Health and Disease,* which found patients who were treated with nonsynthetic cannabinoids were up to three times more likely to report at least a 30 percent reduction in chronic neuropathic pain compared with a placebo.

Lupus

This is another case where cannabis might possibly be a way to help manage some of the symptoms of this autoimmune disease, if not the actual condition itself. "Cannabis can help relieve the pain and inflammation that can be common among patients with lupus," says Brown. "It is possible that cannabinoids can act as an immuno-suppressant, which is beneficial to combat the hyperactive immune system that accompanies [the condition]."

Menstrual Cramps

Depending on the source of the cramps, Brown notes, a treatment that includes a combination of high CBD and broad-spectrum low THC could help to ease the cramping pain and discomfort. Meanwhile, Chasen suggests the use of vaginal suppositories with a 1:1 CBD to THC ratio for more immediate relief, although "consuming through other routes of administration, like oral or inhalation, may also be helpful," she notes.

Migraines

Hormonal migraines "are best targeted with CBD and CBG together," according to Brown. "THC can sometimes make the condition worse. If migraines are caused from stress, then a combination of THC and CBD may be a good option."

Multiple Sclerosis

When it comes to neurodegenerative diseases like multiple sclerosis, CBD and CBG are both apparently "showing promise in slowing the progression" of those conditions, Brown explains. In addition, she says, "reduction in anxiety and improved sleep are commonly reported with cannabis use amongst MS patients."

N

Nausea

"This is one of the few ailments cannabis can conclusively help with," says Chasen. Whether it's dealing with the loss of appetite in HIV/AIDS patients or the aftereffects of chemotherapy, cannabis is now viewed by many as a legitimate form of relief due to the way it can ease nausea. "Inhaled cannabis rich in THC, CBD and THC8 can offer immediate relief of nausea from various causes," says Brown. This is why Clifton credits cannabis with being a significant factor for the decline in deaths from HIV/AIDS.

O

Obesity ▶

Ironically, while experts believe cannabis can help increase appetite for those suffering from anorexia or the aftereffects of chemotherapy, it might also be able to help curb obesity. Says Chasen, "THC, CBD and limonene...have shown anorexic effects and may be able to reduce appetite." Adds Brown, "Cannabinoids can help regulate the nervous system. Preclinical studies demonstrate that THCV can act as an appetite suppressant, so strains rich in it are great to avoid the common 'munchies' side effect of cannabis use."

P

Parkinson's Disease

The good news is that there has been a lot of information gathered about the relationship between cannabis and Parkinson's, according to Clifton. The not-so-good news? Clifton says that in half of the cases studied, cannabis didn't help slow the tremors that are associated with the condition. Meanwhile, Chasen suggests that FECO—a full-spectrum alcohol preparation with a high concentration of CBD—"may be able to dramatically reduce tremors." Either way, don't dismiss cannabis as a way to help. "Even in situations where the tremors weren't reduced, patients reported an improvement in symptoms," Clifton says. "They think it's because cannabis manages the anxiety and sleep disorders around Parkinson's." Brown adds that "the entourage effect of cannabinoids, specifically those high in CBG, can help to diminish neurodegeneration. Often, patients are finding reduction in spasticity with inhaled cannabis."

Psoriasis

This is something that Clifton says she takes personally because "I have horrible skin. It was almost too much to live in when I was younger, and I had a standing appointment once a month with dermatologists." CBD in the form of topicals has definitely provided relief. In addition, according to Brown, "oral administration of full-spectrum cannabis, including CBD:THC:CBC, has shown tremendous potential in reducing the frequent flare-ups psoriasis patients experience."

Quick Tip

Start with small doses of a tincture with a higher CBD-to-THC ratio if you don't want to experience the psychoactive effects of medical marijuana.

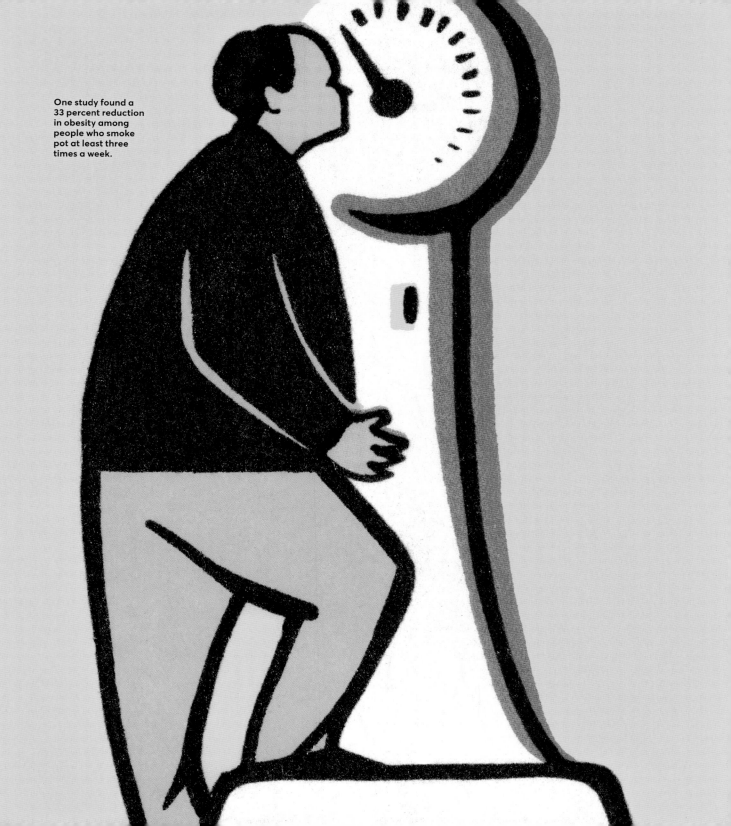

One study found a 33 percent reduction in obesity among people who smoke pot at least three times a week.

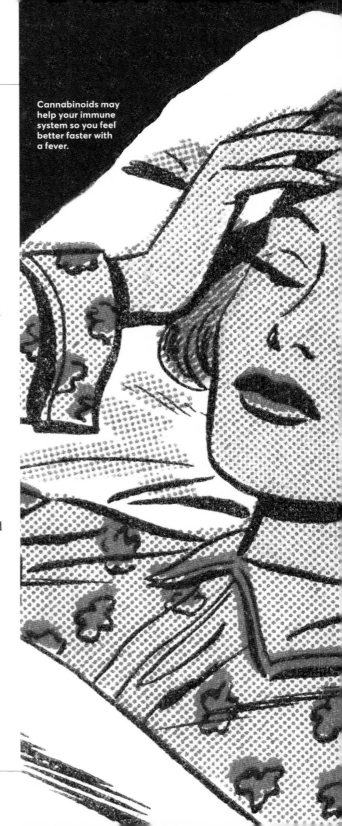

Cannabinoids may help your immune system so you feel better faster with a fever.

Q Fever ▶

According to the Mayo Clinic, this is a bacteria-driven infection that causes flu-like symptoms and can be transmitted to humans through animals, particularly barnyard animals like goats, cows and sheep. At this time, there is no direct research delving into how cannabis use might provide a cure for Q fever. However, as is the case with the flu, using it might improve your immune system enough to fight off an infection or ease the symptoms such as headaches, muscle aches, fatigue and nausea.

Rheumatoid Arthritis

"Because arthritis patients have a higher amount of CB2 receptors in their joints, high CBD:THC ratios such as 30:1 in oral form may offer relief," says Brown. However, don't see cannabis as the only thing you need to add to relieve arthritis pain. Explains Clifton, "Inflammation comes from the inside out," so if you have a poor diet and have been storing up unhealthy fat or you're sleeping less, you leave yourself open to other health problems that can exacerbate your joint aches.

Stroke

There may well be plenty of help to be had here. Brown points out that "cannabinoids are neuroprotective," meaning that the antioxidant properties of CBD and CBG have been "observed to potentially slow brain damage

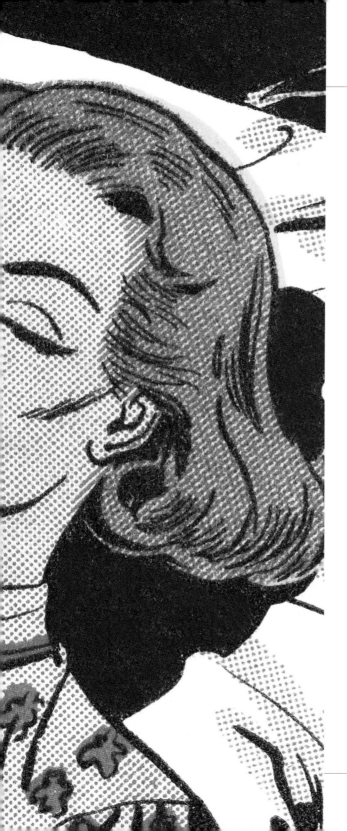

in the aftermath of a stroke that is mostly associated with the increased level of oxidative stress, excitotoxicity and inflammation." Plus, she adds, the anti-inflammatory properties of THC "show promise" when it comes to stroke recovery.

T

Tourette's Syndrome

Brown and Clifton both cite studies done in Germany on the effect of cannabis on children with Tourette's. While the results seem to indicate that THC "could increase obsessive-compulsive disorder behavioral tendencies" that are often associated with Tourette's, says Brown, "high CBD and low THC–20:1–would be the recommendation" for possible treatment. Clifton does say that in one German study, one child's Tourette's got inexplicably worse while he was using cannabis. However, "they circled back, and it turned out he'd quit using it and was using alcohol to control his symptoms. As soon as he stopped using that and began using cannabis again, he got better."

U

Ulcerative Colitis

Not unlike Crohn's disease and other conditions involving the stomach, there is the possibility of pain relief from cannabis for sufferers of ulcerative colitis. There are "abundant CB2 receptors in the lower abdominal organs," explains Brown, and they can potentially respond very well to a treatment involving a combination of CBD and CBG.

Vascular Disease

While research in humans is still in progress, animal studies have shown that CBD may help protect against vascular damage caused by a diet that's high in glucose. It's also been shown to have a direct impact on isolated arteries, helping to reduce vascular tension when administered in animal models. And CBD's anti-inflammatory properties may play a role in reducing tissue damage that can occur after a period of ischemia (lack of oxygen to the heart). While researchers caution that more studies are necessary, investigators say it appears that CBD plays a positive role in treatment in supporting the peripheral and cerebral vasculature.

Wasting Syndrome

Also called "cachexia," this is a symptom of many chronic conditions such as HIV/AIDS, chronic renal failure, multiple sclerosis and cancer. It causes extreme weight loss and wasting away of muscles. Brown says that there have been cases where THC and THC8 have been used to combat cachexia.

Fragile X Syndrome ▶

Many children who are diagnosed with fragile X syndrome—a genetic condition that causes a range of developmental problems—also typically experience behavioral issues like anxiety, hyperactive behavior, attention deficit disorder and autism spectrum disorder. Early research indicates that a pharmaceutical CBD gel from Zynerba Pharmaceuticals may significantly improve behavioral symptoms in children and adolescents who have been diagnosed with the syndrome.

Yeast Infection

Similar to the situation with jock itch, according to Clifton, using a medicine that contains pinenes may take care of the inflammation that often leads to yeast infections. Brown also says that "there is a possibility of CBD and CBG showing promise due to their antifungal and antibacterial properties. This does not include the inhalation mode."

Zoster

This virus, known to cause shingles as well as chicken pox, can bring on serious pain and typically affects older adults. It can be notoriously difficult to treat, according to Clifton, but cannabis can potentially modulate the agony, because it is what she refers to as "neuropathic." "I would take something orally, a product containing THC, because it can work deep in the tissue" where inflammation is occurring, she advises.

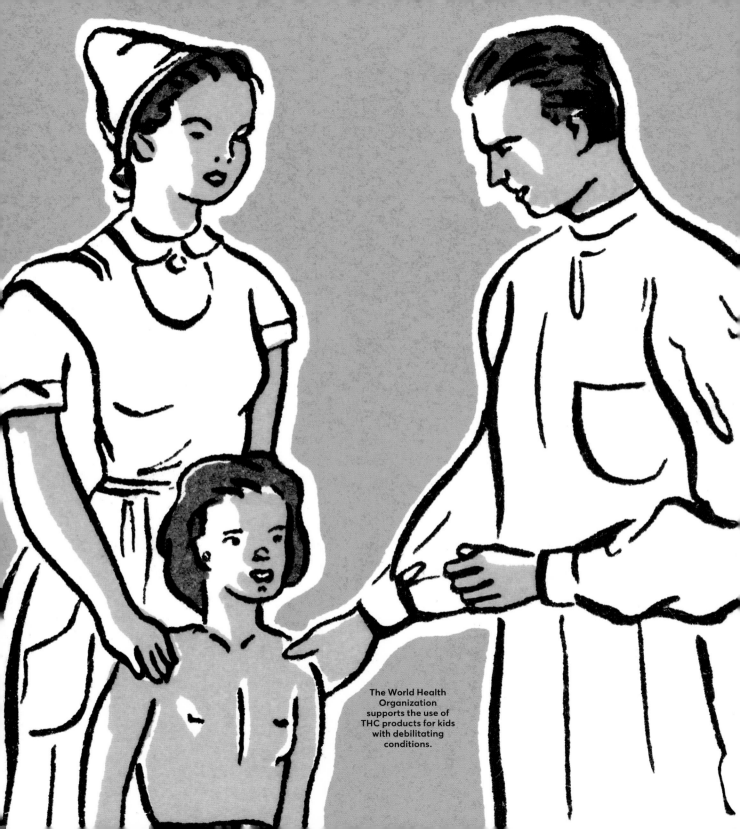

The World Health Organization supports the use of THC products for kids with debilitating conditions.

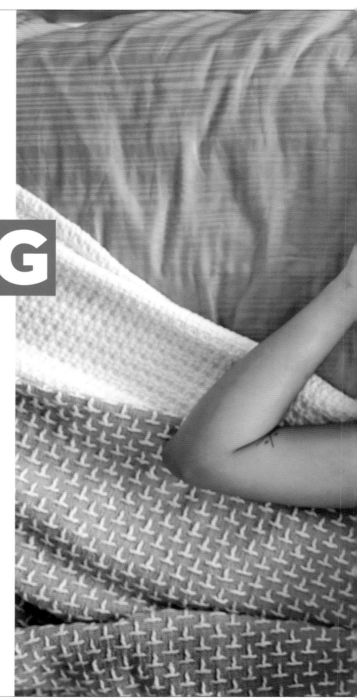

YOU ARE GETTING SLEEPY

SCIENTISTS SAY THE COMPOUNDS IN CANNABIS CAN HELP YOU GET MORE Zs.

Years before CBD became the big thing in cannabis, users were happy to light up before bed and cruise off to a luxuriously stoned sleep. The THC in cannabis, people assumed, helped them get a solid seven or eight hours of un-interrupted dozing.

Now, some companies are hyping CBD–containing no THC–as a cure for insomnia. But is that accurate?

"There's a lot of sedation people can get from CBD," says Mary Clifton, MD, an internal medicine physician based in New York. "Even though we say CBD is not

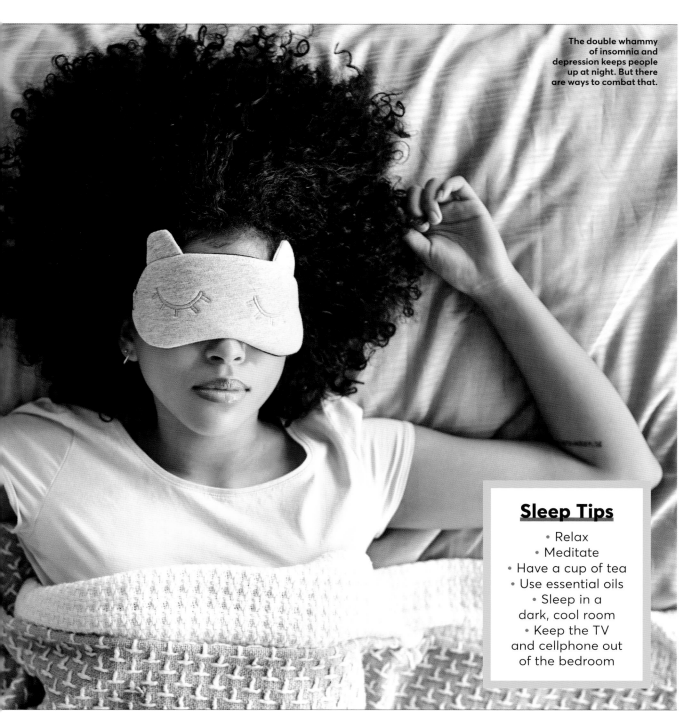

The double whammy of insomnia and depression keeps people up at night. But there are ways to combat that.

Sleep Tips

- Relax
- Meditate
- Have a cup of tea
- Use essential oils
- Sleep in a dark, cool room
- Keep the TV and cellphone out of the bedroom

psychoactive, it clearly is. It works in the brain, particularly in seizure disorders, and it helps control a lot of anxieties for a lot of people. There's a definite effect in the central nervous system with CBD. Most people can get quite an improvement of a sleep disorder with just CBD. If that doesn't work, you can add THC."

According to the projectcbd.org website, "Cannabinoids have been used for centuries to promote sleepiness and help people stay asleep. Among medical-marijuana patients, 48 percent report using cannabis to help with insomnia." The site also reports that CBD "is alerting or mildly stimulating in moderate doses...while its psychoactive counterpart delta-9-tetrahydrocannabinol (THC) tends to be sedating. Both can be alerting or sedating, depending on dosage."

Laura Lagano, a New Jersey-based integrative and functional medicine nutritionist and author of *The CBD Oil Miracle*, agrees with that assessment. "For insomnia, CBD alone can be helpful for some people," she explains. "For others, CBD plus a tiny bit of THC can be better. Because of its biphasic response, CBD typically has a stimulating effect at lower doses and a sedating effect at higher doses."

■ DOs AND DON'TS OF DOSING

"Some of my patients are getting great results from starting dosages," Clifton notes, citing individual levels of CB receptors and lifestyle factors, such as diet and exercise, that all play roles in how the substance will affect a person. "So one person may need a very high dose to get the desired outcome, whereas somebody else just needs a lot less."

Non-cannabinoid terpenes—organic compounds found in plants—are also a factor, adds Clifton. "People understate the value of the terpenes in the

About 50 to 70 million people in the U.S. suffer from chronic long-term sleep disorders each year."

NATIONAL INSTITUTES OF HEALTH

formulas they're using," she says. "You can surround the THC or CBD you're using with a smart variety of terpenes that will handle specifically what you're trying to control. You're basically surrounding your CBD with essential oils. A lot of terps have an overlap with the essential oil community. If you don't have a wide variety of cannabis choices, you could look to lavender for relaxation. Avoid the citruses because those can be stimulating. For instance, limonene might be something to avoid before bed. A quick search online might help you clarify which terps you want to try, or what different essential oils you might want to try around your CBD."

Clifton cites a 2018 PTSD study by the British Columbia Centre for Substance Use that found "criminally insane patients whose sleep was limited to five hours a night and had nightmares up to five nights a week improved considerably with a formulation that included CBD and THC—by two hours a night, from five to seven, and decreased the frequency of the nightmares from five to one a week."

A 2019 CBD study of 72 patients conducted by the Wholeness Center in Fort Collins, Colorado, however, concluded that the patients "demonstrated a more sustained response to anxiety than for sleep over time." The researchers reported that "sleep scores improved within the first month in 48 patients (66.7 percent), but fluctuated over time" and found that "high-dose CBD at 160 mg increased the duration of sleep."

Clifton insists that patients only use CBD or other sleep aids sporadically. "It's better if you can avoid taking it every night," she says. "I generally encourage people to take a sleep aid for no more than two or three nights a week and try to get by on good sleep

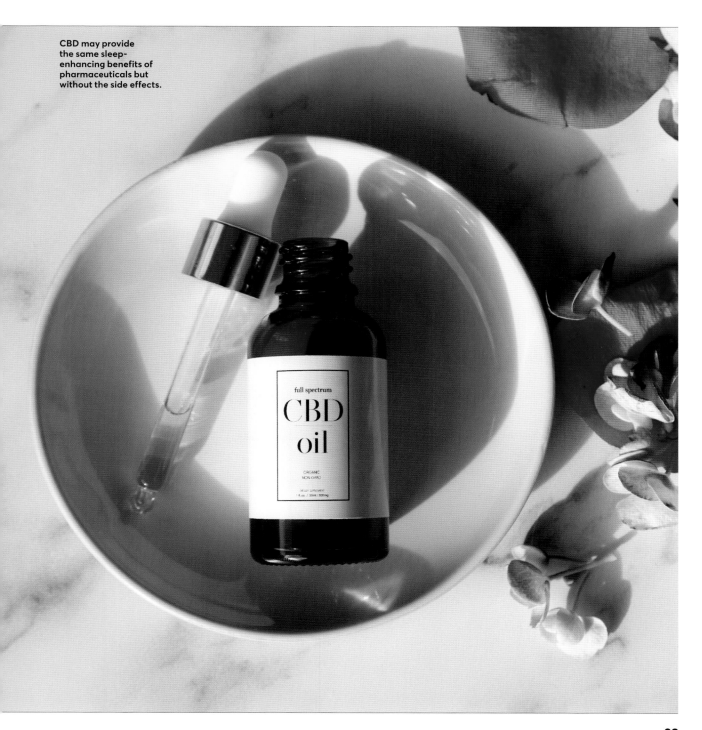

CBD may provide the same sleep-enhancing benefits of pharmaceuticals but without the side effects.

hygiene the rest of the nights. Maybe use it on the nights when you have something you really need to be present for the next day. That way you can allow it to work for you for longer.

"I realize that some people have a lot of difficulty sleeping," Clifton acknowledges. "Taking a sleep aid every night is something that some people need." And despite the Wholeness Center study results, Clifton's experience suggests CBD might be a good sleep solution long term. "I haven't seen the benefit of CBD wear off as quickly as other products like Ambien" she says.

■ GOOD SLEEP HYGIENE HELPS, TOO

When beginning to experiment with the sleep benefits of CBD, Clifton recommends starting with commonsense sleep hygiene tips, like keeping the bedroom dark, cool and quiet, and getting enough exercise during the day. She suggests avoiding edibles in the beginning, because it is harder to control the dose. "I always recommend that people start with a smoke or a vape [see page 38 on the ins and outs of vaping and the current lung issues people are facing] or a tincture when you're learning how to use the product to see if it's working. It's going to take several doses. The titration is going to take two weeks. In most studies, when people are successful they're given two weeks to titrate their dose. I tell people to take a dose and set an alarm on their phone and see how they feel 20 minutes later. The people who start out with edibles just don't have success. They don't get a result quickly enough, they can't assess if it's working or not, they don't know when to take a second dose, and they end up saying it doesn't work for them."

So no on edibles; yes on higher doses and adding THC to the CBD; make sure you learn about terpenes; be conscious of your sleep hygiene; and don't overdo it on the medication. If you follow this advice, you should be out like a light for a solid sleep most nights–which sure beats walking the halls at 4:20 a.m.

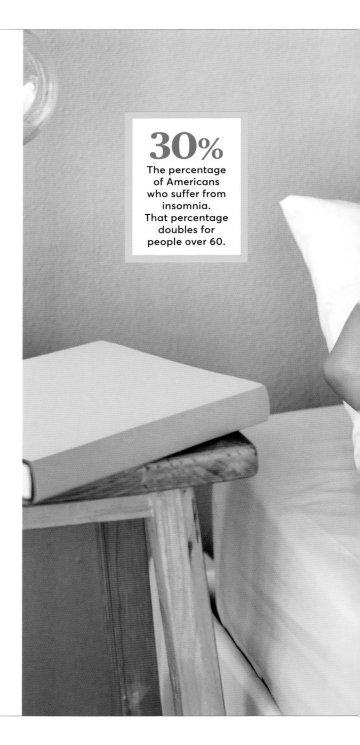

30%
The percentage of Americans who suffer from insomnia. That percentage doubles for people over 60.

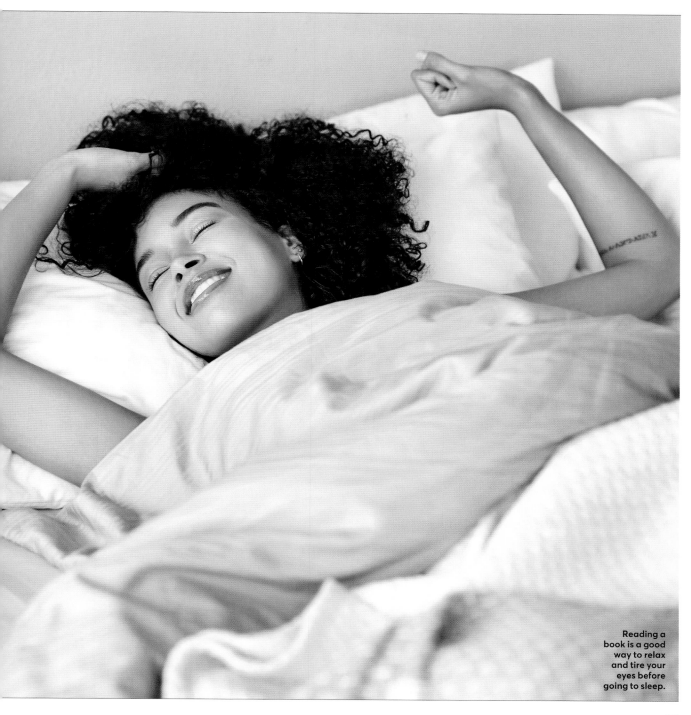

Reading a book is a good way to relax and tire your eyes before going to sleep.

GETTING BACK IN ACTION

HOW I LEARNED TO STOP WORRYING AND TRY MEDICAL MARIJUANA FOR MY BACK PAIN.

It's safe to say, I'm not a particularly adventurous person when it comes to drugs. I've smoked marijuana three times in my entire life (and inhaled only once). When my friends in college would light up, I'd suddenly remember an important meeting I had to get up early for. And I don't think I've ever watched two minutes of a Cheech & Chong movie.

Growing up, I'd seen the antidrug PSAs. I'd read the news. I saw footage from Woodstock. In my mind, taking a single hit off a lone joint would leave me trying to take my pants off over my head while hijacking a truck filled with Twinkies. Pot was the devil's plant. Therefore, those who used it were evil as well. Even as public opinion shifted and marijuana—at least the medical version—became socially acceptable, I've resisted trying it, courtesy of my irrational fear. Then I heard from my 80-something mom, who said she'd started using CBD oil for her arthritis, which she was

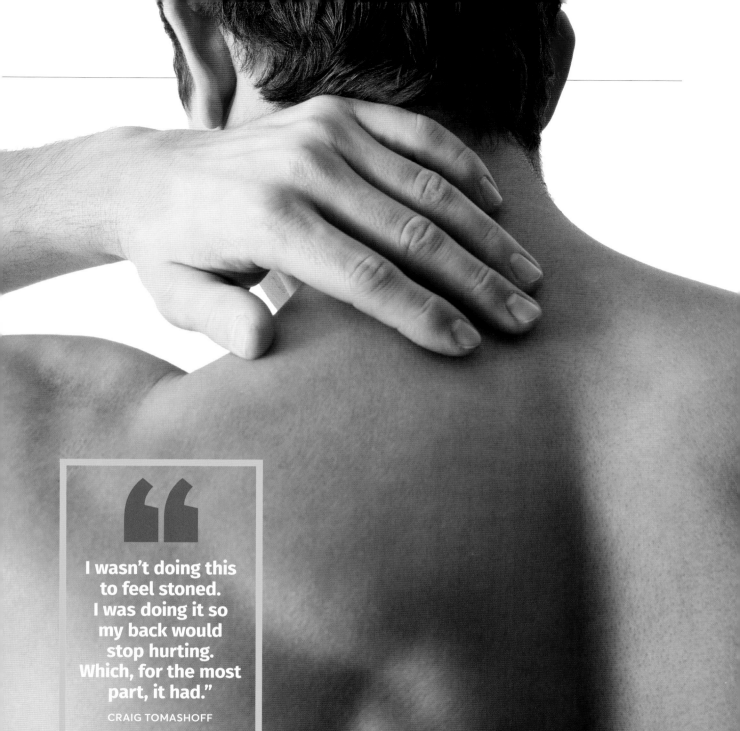

> **"I wasn't doing this to feel stoned. I was doing it so my back would stop hurting. Which, for the most part, it had."**
>
> CRAIG TOMASHOFF

doing after my brother had started using it for his chronic back pain.

Suddenly, I had no excuse. If the ultraconservative family that taught me drug use was wrong now saw cannabis as an acceptable treatment, I probably should too. And I could use the help. I've had some major sciatica issues for years now, probably the curse of making a living by sitting at a computer for hours every day. My back had become so painful that when walking my dog, I often had to stop to lie on the ground and do yoga stretches just to make it back home.

▪ FIGHTING THE FEAR

Surgery and drugs were certainly an option, but frankly, they scared me as much as the sight of a bong. Via a fellow writer's recommendation, I contacted a Colorado company, Infinite CBD (infinitecbd.com). The marketing director, Ali Munk, explained that Infinite had a wide range of hemp-derived CBD products for beginners like me. She reassured me that the products didn't require my getting a medical card and wouldn't provide that Twinkie-munching high I was worried about. Within a week, I received a goody box filled with CBD gummies, drops, oils and lotions, plus a vaping pen.

I set all this out on my desk and then...stared at it for two weeks, still worried that using any of it would leave me couch-bound and craving Cheetos and Grateful Dead music. My kids were tremendously amused that their non-drug-user dad had this little "stash," mocking me for how nervous I got just talking about it, which was the incentive I needed to finally give in and try CBD.

Bearing in mind Munk's advice that dosing is tricky and to start slow to find what works, I boldly ate one 25 mg gummy. And instantly spit it out. Perhaps it was just my fear manifesting as the taste of mowed grass, but my superior gag reflex took charge. After waiting a few minutes (and feeling a sense of failure), I tried again. This time, the gummy stayed down. I'd been warned it'd take up to 90 minutes to feel any relief. Two hours later, though, my back was still throbbing.

> **Within a few minutes of applying each product, I was better. I swear, it stopped feeling like there was a minivan sitting on top of my lower vertebrae. It was now, at best, a Vespa."**
>
> CRAIG TOMASHOFF

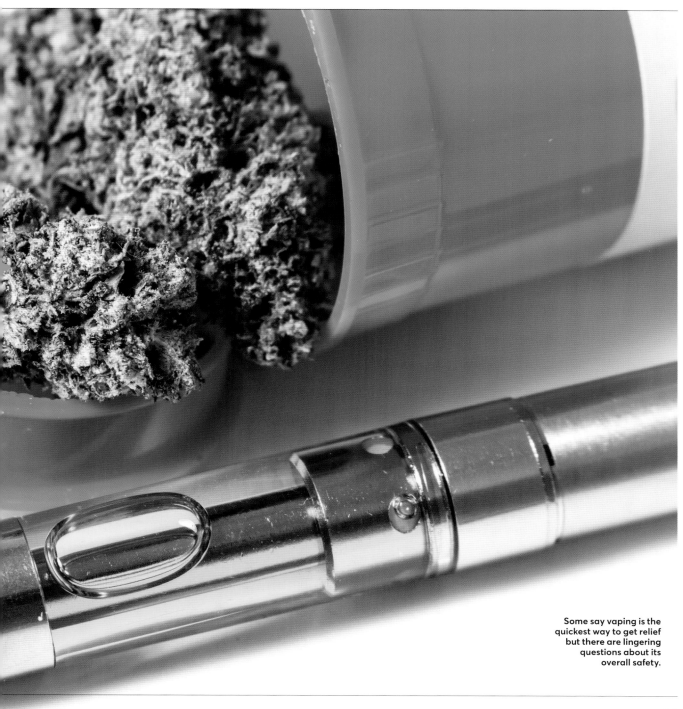

Some say vaping is the quickest way to get relief but there are lingering questions about its overall safety.

Determined to try again, the next night, I tried one-and-a-half gummies. And 90 minutes in, I still felt nothing. At first, this left me discouraged, until I realized...feeling nothing is the point! I wasn't doing this to feel stoned. I was doing it so my back would stop hurting. Which, for the most part, it had. There was still a dull ache, but nothing as intense at it sometimes gets. Perhaps it was a fluke, but this was enough to get me to try again the next night.

This time I went for Infinite's Pineapple Express Isolate Dropper. Munk had suggested trying eight to 10 drops under my tongue, to help relax me and curb my back inflammation. Sadly, about three drops in, I mistakenly swallowed everything instead of letting it sit. It tasted like a glass of liquefied pine needles–so, like the first round of gummies, I spit everything out. One night later, I tried again and, this time, managed to get my 10 drops in with no problem. Still, I had to resort to Aleve and a heating pad to curb my backache.

I tried a third time the next evening and again wondered why I wasn't feeling different. Then I tried to get up from the couch to get a glass of water and suddenly realized: I didn't really want to move. My back...hell, all of me...felt more relaxed and comfortable. Maybe it was wishful thinking. Or maybe the drops were actually relieving my pain. Either way, I was happy with the result.

◼ TO VAPE OR NOT TO VAPE

Next up, I began using Infinite's Freezing Point cream and salve, rubbing both liberally into my lower back three or four times a day. This was by far the easiest way to use CBD, because (a) there was nothing for me to gag on, and (b) it literally is no different from rubbing on some BenGay–only without that overpowering smell. Within a few minutes of applying each product, I was better. I swear, it stopped feeling like there was a minivan sitting on top of my lower vertebrae. It was now, at best, a Vespa.

Which brings me to the last item, the vape pen. While eating a gummy or rubbing on a lotion didn't feel like I was doing something immoral, that's exactly how vaping seemed. Still, I'd promised myself I'd try everything, so I followed Munk's directions, fired the pen up and inhaled as deeply as I could.

◼ A SNEAKY SENSE OF RELIEF

I was expecting to expel that same cloud of vapor we've all seen coming from the tattooed, bearded hipster dude who pulls up next to you at a red light. Instead, though, there was just a pine-flavored burning sensation drifting into my throat. Every expert I'd interviewed for this article insisted vaping is by far the quickest way to get CBD relief. Fifteen minutes in, though, the only thing that had me feeling worse than the twinge in my back was the lingering cough from inhaling the pen.

I was all set to write about how disappointed I was that vaping didn't affect me at all. Then, once again, I realized relief had snuck up on me. I'd gone an hour without having to stretch out my back or grab the heating pad. I actually felt comfortable, just as I (eventually) had with the gummies, drops and lotions. All I could do was wonder why I'd waited so long for this relief.

Years of anti-pot propaganda had me expecting to become Jeff Bridges in *The Big Lebowski*, so I couldn't accept that that's not what medical marijuana is. It's about getting pain relief, not getting the munchies. Sure, CBD (and maybe a modicum of THC) alone won't cure anyone. It won't help everyone. If you want to heal back pain without opioids and surgery, stretching and exercise are as critical as cannabis-based remedies. Still, ruling out medical marijuana because you can't shake those visions of reefer madness makes no sense.

I may wake up in pain tomorrow, bent over as if I'm about to ring the bell at Notre Dame. Or I may go for a 3-mile dog walk with a smile on my face. Either way, I will be more confident, knowing that I didn't let irrational fear rule my life. I stepped outside my little world, which left me feeling pretty good–spiritually, as well as in my lower back.

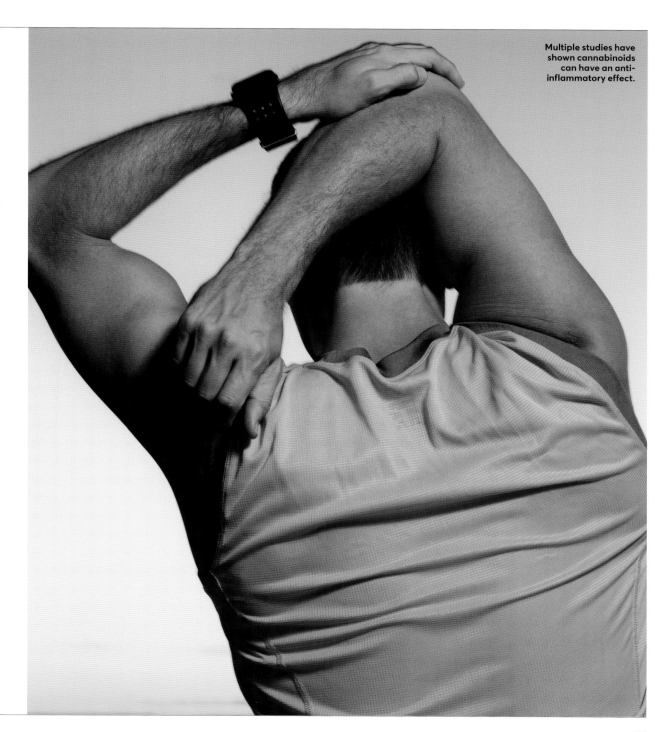

Multiple studies have shown cannabinoids can have an anti-inflammatory effect.

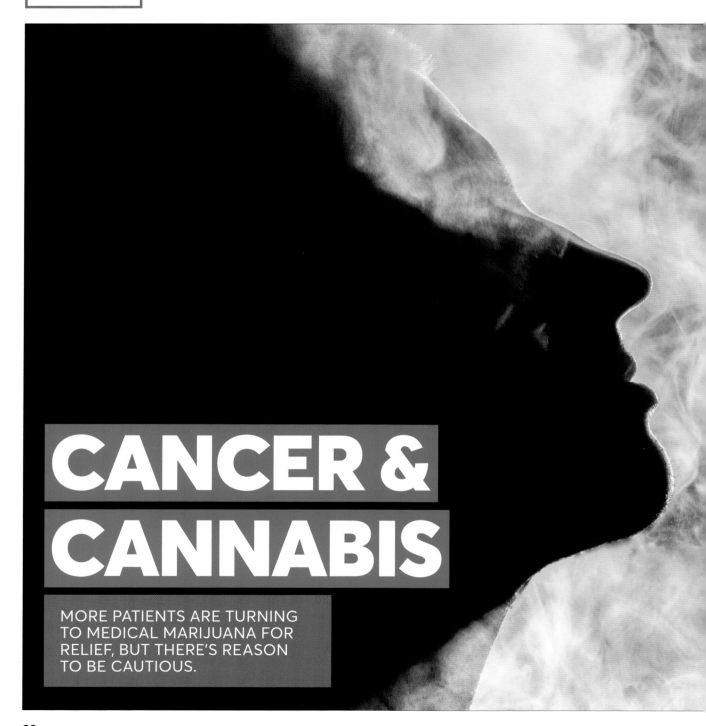

CANCER & CANNABIS

MORE PATIENTS ARE TURNING TO MEDICAL MARIJUANA FOR RELIEF, BUT THERE'S REASON TO BE CAUTIOUS.

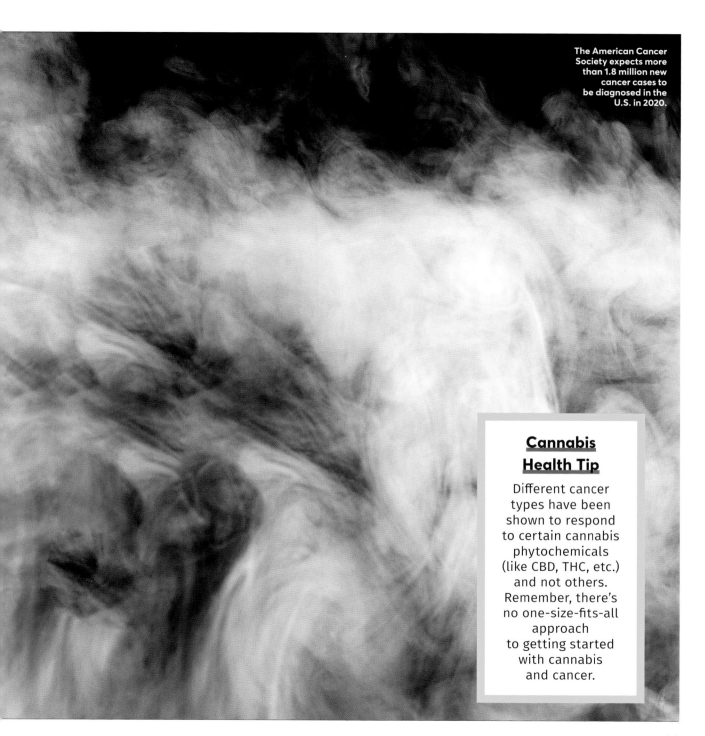

The American Cancer Society expects more than 1.8 million new cancer cases to be diagnosed in the U.S. in 2020.

Cannabis Health Tip

Different cancer types have been shown to respond to certain cannabis phytochemicals (like CBD, THC, etc.) and not others. Remember, there's no one-size-fits-all approach to getting started with cannabis and cancer.

The number is almost too startling to process—nearly 40 percent of all Americans will be diagnosed with cancer at some point in their lives, according to the National Cancer Institute. That's roughly 100,000,000 people, which virtually guarantees that if you don't experience it yourself, you'll have a loved one who does. Given the broad reach of the disease, and the fact that there are more than 100 different types of cancer, it makes sense that patients have started looking beyond the traditional medical treatments to find relief. It's a search that is increasingly including marijuana.

"A diagnosis of cancer is terrifying, and when conventional therapies such as chemotherapy and radiation therapy carry a 2 percent survival rate five years post-treatment (in some cases), it's no surprise that people are considering other therapy options," says Rachel Knox, MD, a cannabinoid medicine specialist at American Cannabinoid Clinics in Portland, Oregon. "For some, one of those options is cannabis."

There is scientific evidence that using this plant is catching on. In a study of more than 800 adults with cancer between 2005 and 2014, the U.S. National Health and Nutrition Examination Survey determined that 40 percent of cancer patients had used marijuana within the previous year to treat symptoms of cancer. That's slightly higher than the rate of marijuana use by adults without cancer, which was 38 percent. Meanwhile, the use of prescription opioids by cancer patients remained stable.

The wave of states legalizing medical marijuana while the survey was conducted and since it was completed likely played a role in the increasing interest in cannabis as a cancer treatment. According to one of the study's co-authors, Jona Hattangadi-Gluth, MD, the legalization of medical marijuana has been associated with a decline in hospitalizations for opioid abuse or dependence. Therefore, cannabis treatments might not only help with the effects of cancer—they might also reduce opioid-related illnesses and deaths.

◼ RELIEVING SEVERAL SYMPTOMS

"Cannabis is less addictive and less harmful than opioids," Knox explains. "On a scale of one to 10, one being least addictive and harmful and 10 being most addictive and harmful, cannabis lands around one and opioids around 10. Also, it's important to note that the data suggests that concomitant use of cannabis with opioids, where necessary, results in a decreased addiction to opioids, decreased desensitization to opioids and improved control over pain with lower doses of opioids."

While there is no scientific evidence that medical marijuana can cure any form of cancer, Knox notes that there is a growing consensus "that it does help manage a variety of symptoms common to cancer or cancer therapie, such as anxiety, depression, poor appetite, insomnia, nausea and vomiting, headaches and migraines, and more."

At the top of the list, though, is the growing belief that using various forms of marijuana can help patients suffering from a variety of maladies manage their pain. That is certainly the case when it comes to cancer. Yet despite marijuana's growing popularity as a form of treatment, Knox urges cancer patients to try a couple of other steps before leaping into any marijuana-based medicines.

"First things first: What's paramount for a patient with cancer to consider is their lifestyle, nutrition being most important," says Knox, whose clinic consults with patients from all across the country. "Before considering cannabis, a patient must convert to a natural, whole-food diet—such as a traditional or plant-based ketogenic diet—and remove any and all toxic exposures from their environment."

In addition, Knox insists that any patient with cancer who is considering cannabis therapy should also consult with a health-care provider knowledgeable in endocannabinology and cannabinoid pharmacology. The danger is that cannabis can interact with other pharmaceutical drugs, which means it should be taken with the supervision of a medical professional who can assist with medication management.

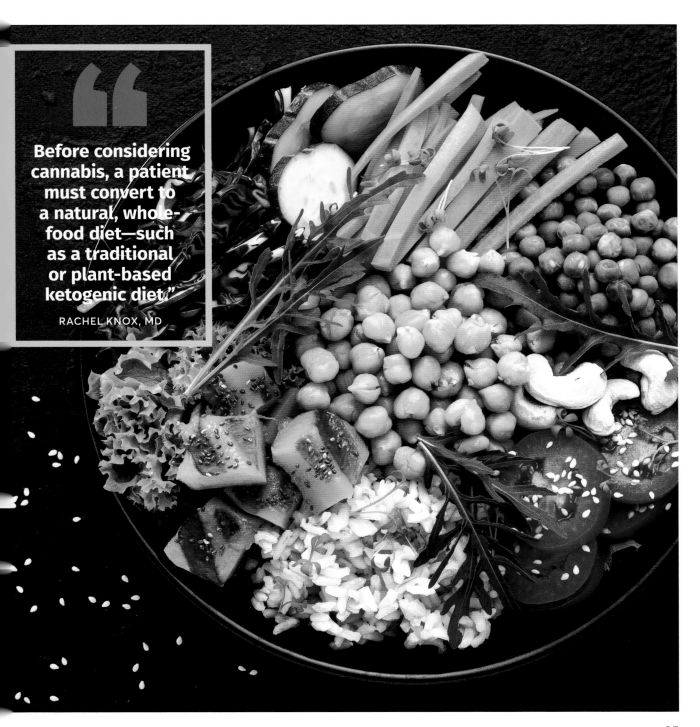

> **Before considering cannabis, a patient must convert to a natural, whole-food diet—such as a traditional or plant-based ketogenic diet."**
>
> RACHEL KNOX, MD

COMFORT AFTER CHEMO

A BREAST CANCER SURVIVOR FINDS HELP AND HOPE WITH CANNABIS.

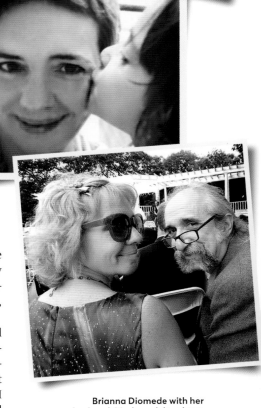

Brianna Diomede with her husband, Mark, and daughters Melody and Azalea (top); sharing a tender moment with Melody (center) and with Mark (bottom).

May 9, 2012, is seared in my memory. That's the day I was diagnosed with a very aggressive collection of tumors in my chest. I was in the shower, and I felt a lump in my armpit. I knew that something wasn't right and went to see my gynecologist right after work (I was an embroiderer at a small factory in Brick Township, New Jersey). He found another tumor in my breast. Mammograms and ultrasounds found two more. On May 22, before removing the tumors, I began a very aggressive

chemotherapy protocol for five months, to bomb my entire body to destroy any growth and eliminate any possibility of stage 4, which is terminal.

When I had to go through all that chemotherapy while having to work and raise two children, my immediate thought was, Let's load up on the weed. I had smoked before I got sick and saw how cannabis had helped a few friends who were dealing with cancer. The difference now is that I don't really get high, I just feel better. It allows me to feel normal. It became a whole new thing for me after cancer. I don't remember what it was like before, when it was fun. Now it's a necessity.

Chemo made me feel like a toxic bomb went off in my body–and when you're trying to deal with the side effects and the whole stress of having cancer, marijuana just takes away everything. I would use it to eat, to sleep, to feel like I could get out of bed and move, but the main thing was the nausea. I was working nine-hour days, so when I got home, I was absolutely taxed. My bones hurt, and cannabis was the only thing that worked. It makes you step out of your head first, then it relieves your symptoms. It's hard to describe–but you definitely leave your body.

After all the chemo, on November 9, I had a bilateral mastectomy and a lymph-node dissection with reconstruction. I then had to undergo 25 days of radiation, just to make sure all the cancer was eradicated. It was like, burn the forest down. But the radiation caused so much damage, I had to have five fat-grafting surgeries over the next three years on top of working and trying to be a good mom to my kids. They're my whole world, so it was quite a shock when I got into a little bit of trouble with Child Protective Services (CPS) in 2014.

■ "I'M LIKE A DIFFERENT PERSON"
I had signed up for psychotherapy through the state, because I didn't have any health insurance, and had to get drug-tested because it's a state program. When I came up positive for marijuana, they had to call CPS. They felt really bad, but they had to do it for legal reasons. It was a long, drawn-out mess. My doctor had to write that it was necessary for my treatment because I couldn't really take anything else. CPS is not fun. That was the last thing I needed in my condition.

Needless to say, it was a huge relief when I was finally able to get a medical-marijuana card. I have refused all pharmaceuticals because of the side effects, with the exception of pain meds post-surgeries. When the program was first started in 2010, you had to have a terminal illness, ALS or AIDS, but now it covers PTSD and people with musculoskeletal spasticity, like myself, who were damaged by radiation. I can get the best-quality flower at my dispensary, with all terpenes listed, and CBG/CBD/THC levels to help me find the best strains to get through my day and night, since I live in constant pain.

I have two broken ribs that refuse to heal, but I also have to keep a house going, so cannabis has been my lifesaver for it all. I use it to sleep, eat, create art [for extra income since she's on disability], function, uplift and balance out the stress and anxiety of being limited.

I get an ounce a month, which costs about $300 to $400, but I get a 20 percent discount because I'm on Social Security. It's not cheap, but it's really, really good. Knowing that it's not been sprayed with anything and with the different levels of terpenes, I know what I'm getting. Two of the strains I like are Montana Silvertip, a hybrid for the daytime, and Lavender, an indica for the nighttime. Silvertip is very high in a cannabinoid called CBG, which has been shown to promote bone growth. My ribs don't hurt when I use it.

I smoke about half a dozen bowls during the day and about half that at night. It makes me feel like a human being. My husband will tell you–when it runs out, I'm a different person. It's like not having coffee in the morning. My youngest is too young to know what it is. My oldest is aware of it, but I don't do it in front of her. She understands that it is a medicine. She knows kids in her class who use it, but she realizes there's a medicinal aspect to it. There's no judgment from her.

Marijuana is not addictive, but feeling happy is addictive, feeling relaxed is addictive. I don't see myself ever stopping using it, because I've been hacked apart so many times, there's no going back to normal. I just want it to be legal for everybody who needs it, regardless of income or status, and available at a reasonable price.

–Brianna Diomede

ENDING THE MISERY

LIGHTING UP HELPS ONE MAN DEFEAT THE DARKNESS OF DEPRESSION.

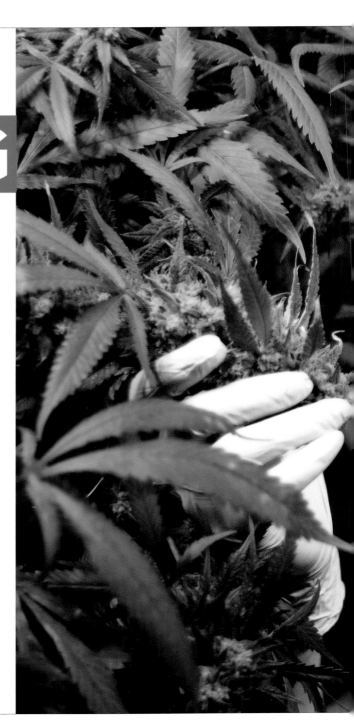

➡ Danny Sloat isn't just the owner of Alpin-stash, one of Colorado's most popular and successful marijuana cultivators. He's also a dedicated patient.

Sloat's cannabis conversion began in 2005, when the Boulder, Colorado, resident was in his early 20s and led a very active life as an avid rock climber, camper and saxophone player. He first experienced a night filled with excruciating stomach pain—and from there, his life became a downward spiral of chronic pain and depression.

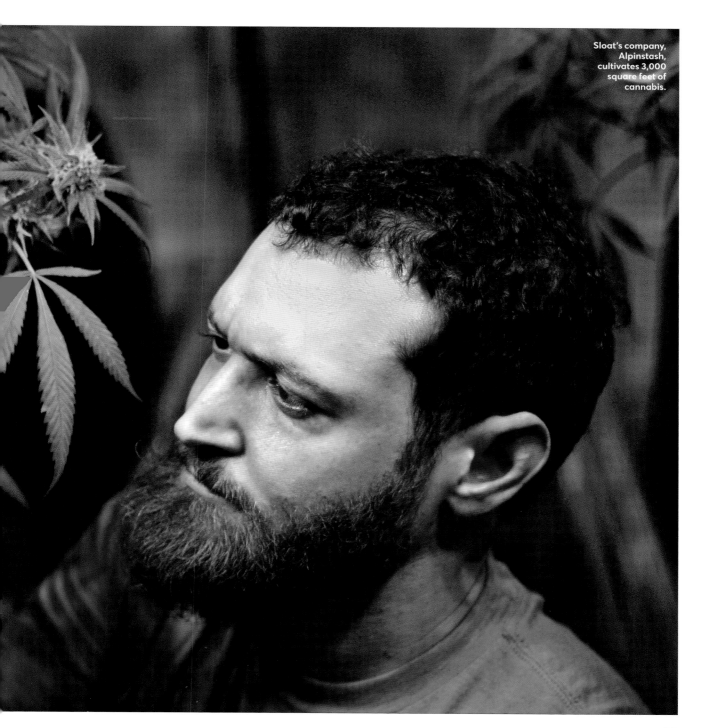

Sloat's company, Alpinstash, cultivates 3,000 square feet of cannabis.

He was diagnosed with a pelvic floor dysfunction–the spasming of the muscles at the bottom of the pelvis–that doctors believed was caused by a hyperactive immune system. (Sloat had suffered from colitis and asthma, conditions that contributed to his pelvic problems, since childhood.)

Despite prescriptions for Antagonin and Vicodin, the stomach pain persisted. Sloat's quality of life began to unravel as he spent the bulk of his time visiting doctors, searching fruitlessly for any help managing his pain. The frustration morphed into depression as Sloat slowly sunk into a funk.

"In fairly short order, I began withdrawing from my friends, withdrawing from social activity... all the while, under very close doctor supervision," he recalls.

Not only were the drugs not helping, they also caused a painful side effect: leaks in other parts of Sloat's body. He was constantly poked and prodded by doctors and given steroid injections and epidurals; trigger-point injections; deep-tissue needling; and needle electrotherapy–but nothing seemed to end his misery.

Seeing no hope for himself, Sloat began letting himself go.

■ "I WAS NOT IN A GOOD SPOT"

"His problems were multiplying, and he had gained 70 pounds–and he's not a big guy," says his father, Jerry, an attorney and cannabis advocate who helped found

The doctor said we can treat the pain with the little hammer or we could use the big hammer... which turned out to be fentanyl. A lollipop and patches of fentanyl."

DANNY SLOAT

Colorado's chapter of the National Organization for the Reform of Marijuana Laws (NORML). "He wouldn't get out of bed. He moved back to our house. He didn't bathe, he didn't shave. He ate junk food when he ate. The only friends he had would come over to steal his drugs. He was no fun to be with, but he had his drugs."

The depression spawned desperation. Says Danny, "The doctor said we can treat the pain with the little hammer, or we could use a big hammer," he says. "By that point, I was very sick of having pain–so I asked for what he

said was the big hammer, which turned out to be fentanyl. A lollipop and patches of fentanyl."

The effects of the fentanyl were devastating. Sloat began sleeping 16 hours a day. He took drugs to wake up and drugs to sleep. Each pill came with its own awful side effect.

"During this time, I developed a nerve impingement syndrome, called thoracic outlet syndrome, in my arm. As my stomach pain faded away, it was replaced by pretty substantial arm pain, numbness, tingling and loss of nerve function," he explains. "So that meant more medications, more injections and things like that." He also had surgery for thoracic outlet, had a rib and muscle removed from his chest and contemplated removing neck muscles as a way to ease the pain.

By 2009, Sloat knew he "was definitely not in a good spot." After being diagnosed with a noncancerous tumor known as acoustic neuroma, he tried to reduce his fentanyl prescription and switched over to OxyContin and Dilaudid. Sloat's doctor told him that his only option at this point was an in-patient facility.

"I was in a really tricky spot, because I wasn't using these painkillers for recreational purposes," he says. "I was in pain...and it was very frustrating, because all I wanted was to not be in pain." That's when Jerry finally stepped in. The elder Sloat suggested his son take advantage of Colorado's new medical cannabis laws to get some relief.

■ LIFTING THE CLOUD OF DEPRESSION

"Once it was legalized, you began to hear about people using it to get benefits," Jerry says. "When I suggested it to Danny, there weren't a lot of alternatives. We'd tried drugs, injections, everything except inpatient. His doctors were not in favor of it. None of the people in the medical profession were in favor it. People said it was a bad drug. We had nothing to lose."

Sloat ingested cannabis via smoking and edibles, and almost immediately, the dark cloud that had hung over him for years began to lift. Not only did cannabis help ease the pain, but "it helped me get out of the negative feedback associated with pain," he says. The nerve activity in his head and arm returned, and his neural activity also increased.

The cannabis also helped Sloat counter the mental fatigue of pain management. He began participating in physical activities once more, which helped him feel like he was living back in the world again.

"It gave him upward momentum and turned his life around completely," Jerry explains. "We were worried that he didn't want to continue living. It had a miraculous effect—it went from black to white. I've never seen that happen to anybody. We spent so much time watching him suffer. I'm just glad that he's happy."

The way Danny Sloat sees it, he essentially owes his life to cannabis. It not only relieved his depression, it gave him a renewed sense of purpose. Which led him to start growing his own plants and eventually launch his own cannabis cultivation company, Alpinstash.

"I had an epiphany. I wanted to focus in the indoor-gardening industry," he says. "The reason I wanted to get out of bed was to take care of these plants. Of course, I want to make money—but for me, growing and caring for these plants is primarily a spiritual pursuit."

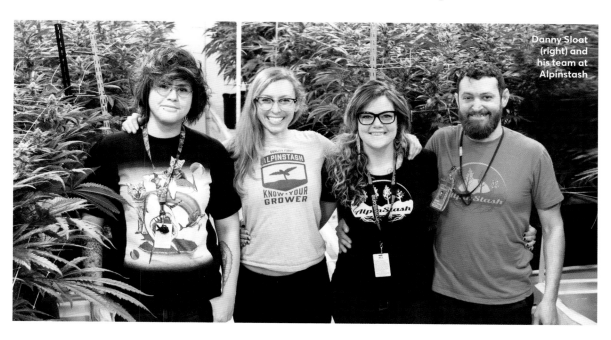

Danny Sloat (right) and his team at Alpinstash

OPTING OUT OF OPIOIDS

OVERWHELMED BY PAINKILLERS, A NURSE FINDS HOPE IN CANNABIS.

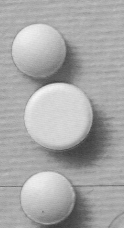

It was pain that drove Debbie Mayberry to become a nurse.

She decided to take up her medical career after losing her newborn son to a congenital heart defect and caring for her grandmother through several health crises. Then, just when she'd achieved her dream of helping her patients get through their agony, she had even more pain to deal with.

In 2011, she slipped and injured her back during a hospital work shift. Suddenly, despite her many years of clinical experience, she wasn't able to nurse herself back to health and a pain-free life. She couldn't work and ended up bedridden, thanks to debilitating pain and depression. Her only source of comfort was a growing array of opioids prescribed for relief.

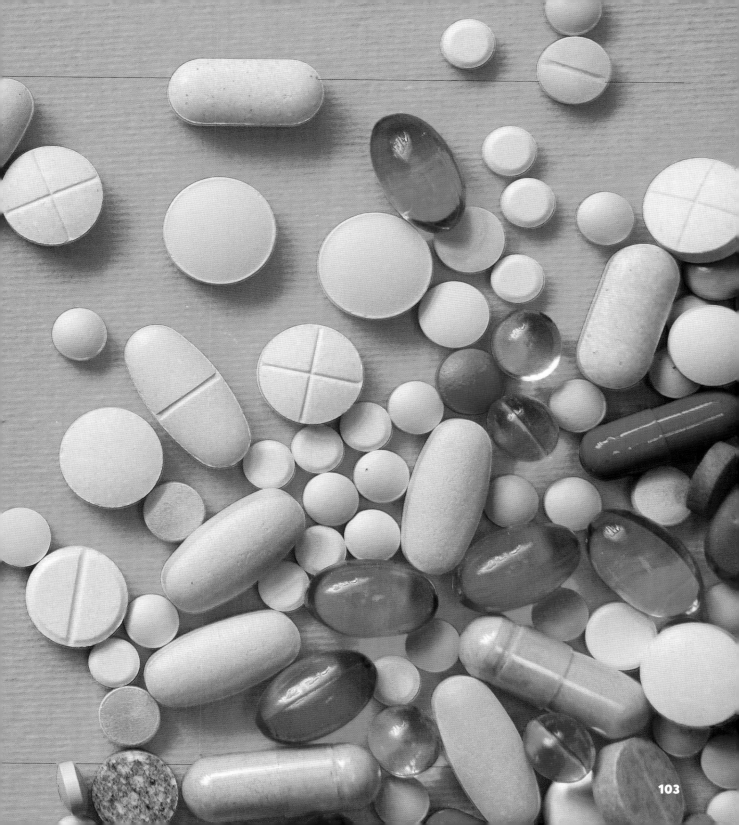

■ OVERWHELMED BY "HORRIBLE" DRUGS

For someone with so much experience dispensing pain meds, Mayberry never saw her own dependency coming. The OxyContin that her workman's-compensation doctor originally prescribed left her unable to function, prompting her to write a scathing letter to him, complaining that "such a horrible drug" left her unable to drive, let alone return to her job.

"He fired me as a patient. He said I was noncompliant. 'If you're not going to take the medication I'm going to prescribe, I can't help you,'" recalls Mayberry.

She then went to her own doctor, who wasn't any more helpful. The physician prescribed Percocet for daily use and advised Mayberry that her nursing career was over. Feeling like she had no other choice, she filed for short- and long-term disability. Things got even worse when she lost her workman's-compensation claim because her preexisting fibromyalgia, not her fall, was seen as the cause of her persistent pain

Mayberry reapplied for short- and long-term disability, and her doctor started prescribing a medicine cabinet of pharmaceuticals: Ativan for sleep; Savella for fibromyalgia; Neurontin for neuropathy;

oxycodone for pain from bulging discs and spinal-nerve-root compression; Effexor for depression. Mayberry began to realize she'd become the sort of painkiller user she would never have let her own patients become. If she missed taking her antidepressants, she flew into uncontrollable rages. After going 36 hours without Ativan because she'd forgotten to get her prescription filled, she recalls being in tears, nonfunctional. "I told my doctor, 'This is seriously not OK. You've got me on all these medications. I'm dependent.'"

Frustrated by her doctor's reluctance to help her ease out of opioid use and uncertain what else was available to treat her condition, Mayberry was desperate. So, when a friend who was using FECO (full-extract cannabis oil) to treat interstitial lung disease suggested in 2014 that Mayberry "stop all that sh-t

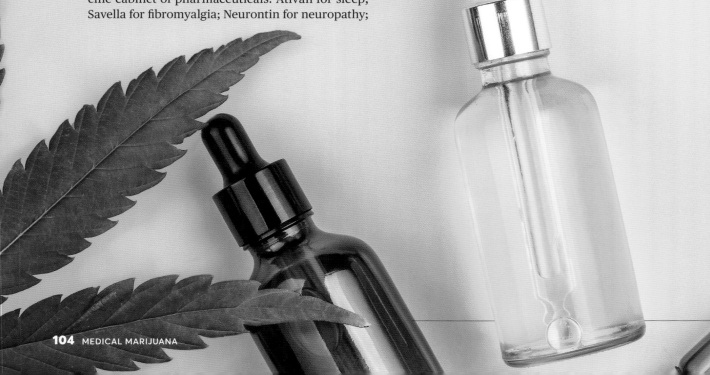

and use cannabis," she decided to give medical cannabis a try. Over the next two years, she slowly but surely began to wean herself from opioid dependency, reclaiming her sanity, health and recovery.

Mayberry began using cannabis oil, putting it in food or taking it in capsule form. "I used all components of the plant, getting a full host of endocannabinoids. It was helping my pain, and it is legal. I was getting my cannabis by doing marijuana-trimming work (for growers); in exchange, they would give me cannabis oil or the cannabis flower—and I could make my own."

◼ SLOW-BUT-STEADY SUCCESS

She soon learned which strains worked for her situation, based on what her growers had available. Some, Mayberry recalls, "were better for getting up and working and having energy and feeling motivated. Others helped me relax at night. They all helped with pain."

But she's discovered that CBD alone isn't enough to ease all that ails her.

"I need the THC because it helps with my mood and helps with my pain," Mayberry explains. "I cook with it. I make infused butter. I smoke as well, when I'm in a place that's appropriate to do that. Even with pharmaceuticals, I always tried to take the least possible so I could participate in life. I wasn't trying to check out. I wanted to participate."

The plan worked. She slowly but surely weaned herself off most of the drugs she'd been taking. "I had tapered down to 10 mg (of oxycodone) or less daily, so I just stopped. My prescription ran out, and I said, 'I'm done.' I was doing really well with pain. I was up and around, able to do things. I still had pain, but I just felt better."

These days, after retiring from nursing, she hopes to become an activist and educator in order to change the public's perception of those in the treatment community, convincing them that cannabis is a healthy, viable alternative to opioids. Says Mayberry, "Change is so slow. I happen to be able to speak up now (about medical marijuana) because I come from a nursing background and can talk with conviction."

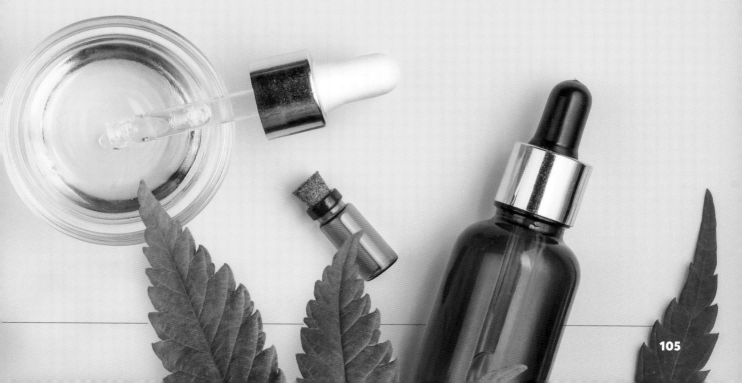

EASING THE TRAUMA

A SURVIVOR OF SEXUAL ASSAULT AND AN IRAQI WAR VET SPEAK OUT ABOUT HOW CANNABIS HAS HELPED RELIEVE THEIR PTSD.

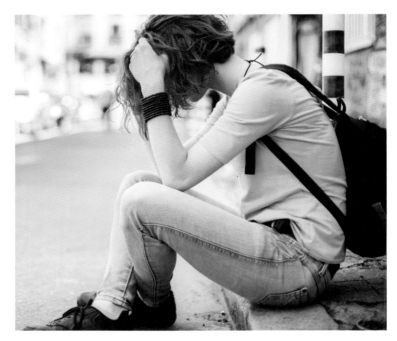

About seven or eight out of every 100 people (or 7 to 8 percent of the population) will be diagnosed with post-traumatic stress disorder (PTSD) at some point in their lives, and about 8 million adults have PTSD during a given year, according to the National Center for PTSD. This is only a small portion of those who have gone through a trauma.

Patients with PTSD can have intense, disturbing thoughts and feelings related to their experience that last long after the traumatic event has ended, with symptoms ranging from flashbacks and nightmares to feelings of extreme sadness, fear or anger. They may avoid situations or people that remind them of the traumatic event, and they may have strong negative reactions to something as ordinary as a loud noise or an accidental touch. Living with PTSD, say patients, is to live with a constant sense of fear or anxiety that gnaws away at their overall well-being.

Much as it can help treat conditions like anxiety, insomnia and pain, cannabis may also play an important role in reducing symptoms of PTSD. Here, two patients share their stories about the role medical marijuana has played in helping them heal.

"CANNABIS GETS ME OUT OF MY HEAD."

One in three women and one in six men in the U.S. will experience sexual violence at some point in their lifetime. Even worse, according to the National Sexual Violence Resource Center, 81 percent of women and 35 percent of men who are victimized by sexual violence also report long- or short-term impacts, such as PTSD. Now, many of these sexual assault survivors are starting to speak out, not only to tell their tragic stories, but also to make it clear that cannabis has helped them manage anxiety attacks and other symptoms of their condition.

No voice is louder than that of sex and relationship coach Ashley Manta, who has become a leading proponent of using medical marijuana to help treat the psychic wounds of sexual assault. After naming her rapist on her blog in 2015, "I had a resurgence of my PTSD, and it was so severe that I quit my full-time job," she explains. "I was having flashbacks and panic attacks. I couldn't eat; I certainly couldn't have sex. Cannabis was the thing that got me through that in ways that my Xanax and antidepressants weren't helping me."

Manta grew up in a relatively conservative environment that taught her cannabis was a drug not to be messed with, but by the time she moved to California in 2013, she was a full-blown cannabis enthusiast.

"California had medical cannabis, so I immediately got my medical card and was able to go into a dispensary," Manta recalls. "There were a plethora of options of consumption methods—and you could find something that was more uplifting, or helped with sleep, or for relieving pain or improving appetite. It was a wonderland."

■ BRINGING A BALANCE

Although researchers continue to look into the connection between cannabis and PTSD, it does stand to reason that the plant can most likely provide some form of relief. After all, sexual abuse and other forms of trauma reportedly alter the communication pathway between the brain and the adrenal glands. That, in turn, can produce excessive amounts of the stress hormone cortisol and potentially lead to everything from increased blood pressure to issues with sleep, digestion and focus. Victims can end up in "fight or flight" mode, depressed and unable to function normally. Meanwhile, studies have found that cannabis can reach out to the body's endocannabinoid system (ECS) to bring the body and the brain back into balance.

That's something Manta experienced firsthand. Not only did cannabis, in conjunction with therapy, help her deal with anxiety attacks related to her PTSD, she also found that cannabis enhanced her sex life, which also then helped elevate her mood. For years, she admits, she experienced pain during intercourse. The only thing that provided relief was Foria Pleasure, a THC-infused lubricant formulated for women.

She's worked as a sex educator for over a decade now, and has decided it's time to start sharing her story with other survivors of sexual assault in order to encourage them to also use cannabis as a way to get their personal lives back together.

"I thought, 'Oh my gosh, there are so many survivors of sexual violence who have this painful experience with sex—they should know about this [treatment],'" Manta explains. "Cannabis, when I vape or smoke it, helps me get out of my head and into my body to be more present."

However, she suggests victims of sexual assault should seek traditonal therapy and not view cannabis as a cure-all. "It's a tool like mindfulness or yoga or meditation...one more thing to have in your tool kit when you're feeling overwhelmed."

"I WAS ABLE TO FIND PEACE."

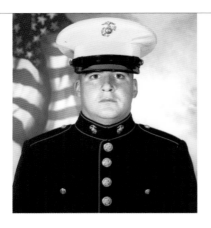

"I was 21 when I enlisted in the Marines in November 2001," recalls Ryan Begin. "I'd just been let go from my job as a heavy-equipment mechanic in Jackman, Maine. It was right after 9/11, so I knew we were going to war; I figured I might as well do my part. A month later, I was headed to boot camp in Parris Island, South Carolina.

As a tow gunner with the 1/2 (1st Battalion, 2nd Marines) Weapons Company, Begin entered Iraq right after the war started in March 2003. "The day we entered, we were in the Battle of An Nasiriyah. We lost 18 guys. Quite a welcome to the combat zone."

Begin was injured in August 2004, when his convoy was on the way back to base, about 45 kilometers south of Baghdad. "I was standing in the turret, manning the tow gun, when a roadside bomb blew my right elbow off and drove me down into the truck. Luckily, there was a corpsman in the back passenger seat, and my arm fell right into his lap. He instantly put on a tourniquet and stuck me with morphine." The only thing holding Begin's arm in place was some skin and some nerves and tendons. The bone had been destroyed. "It was a long ride back to base. I was put in a Blackhawk and taken to Baghdad for surgery before going to Germany and then Bethesda Naval Hospital [now Walter Reed]."

■ "THERE WAS NO GETTING BETTER"

Begin was in Bethesda for a month and a half and had about 35 surgeries before finally going home. "I went from being a warrior to being a broken shovel no one needs. I wondered, 'What the heck is going to happen now?' They had me on every medication you can think of—painkillers, blood-pressure drugs, antidepressants. My psychiatrist put me on Valium; dextroamphetamine, which is a speed; and Seroquel, a sleeping pill. I was basically speed-balling. That was my life."

Begin attempted suicide at least three times between 2005 and 2009. "I was extremely unstable. One time, I took 40 Baclofen; another time, 90 Valium; and another, a bottle of Klonopin. I felt that hopeless. I felt there was no way I could return to the productivity level I had before. There was no getting better." His low point, he says, was when he crashed his truck while drunk and high on painkillers and assaulted the arresting officer. He spent 43 days in jail, most of it in solitary confinement. "I was getting only a portion of my pills and started reading, so my mind kind of reactivated. It allowed me to see that I needed to change—or this was going to be my new home."

Although Begin says aggression was a problem, he dislikes the term PTSD. "I look at it as an identity crisis. You live 21 years of your life a certain way, then you go to a combat zone and have to learn a whole new identity—eliminate the threat—or you're going to be a liability to everyone around you. But when you return to society, you can't eliminate the threat every time there's a stressful situation. You have to change your behavioral pattern for a noncombative society."

One of the ways he made this change, he notes, was "by bringing myself back to zero. I lived on a pig farm with no TV, no nothing, and shoveled pig manure every morning. My arm is fused and is about 8 inches shorter, but I have use of my fingers and can use it as an assist limb."

Another way was to get off the pain medication and rely solely on cannabis for relief. Luckily for Begin, cannabis became medically legal in Maine in 2009–thanks in part to his efforts. "I was involved in the legislation and testifying."

Begin says he is not strain-specific, "but I do like the ones with high THC, more of the Indica hybrids." He smokes 10 to 12 joints a day and uses edibles for sleeping.

■ MAKING ACTIVISM TRANSPARENT

"With PTSD, you're constantly reacting; I find cannabis gives you that second to think instead of just reacting," says Begin. "It allows you to take a breath, to say, 'OK, let's think about this. We're not in Iraq, we're on the streets of Maine. No one is trying to kill you.' It puts you in the now."

But because marijuana is still a Schedule I drug, the VA won't compensate patients for it. So Begin's wife, who also has a medical-marijuana card, and Begin grow 12 plants indoors with 4,000-watt lights. "It's expensive–about $500 a month. There's a light bill, nutrient bill, water bill, plus your time."

Ultimately, Begin hopes others will also be able to find natural relief. "What we need now is transparent activism, if we want to move this forward, If everyone who used cannabis were truly open about it, I don't think we'd be in this dilemma."

VETERANS FAVOR THE USE OF MEDICAL CANNABIS

The American Legion shared the results of a survey of veteran households conducted by an independent public opinion research company regarding the use of cannabis as a treatment for mental and physical conditions. In the survey, 513 respondents identified as veterans, while 289 identified as family members or caregivers of veterans. Both groups showed overwhelming support for medical cannabis.

GROWING SUPPORT FOR TREATMENT

While most respondents do not use cannabis to treat medical conditions or know a veteran who does, most support its use to treat mental or physical conditions.

ABOUT THE RESPONDENTS
Most respondents were more than 45 years old.

78%
Veteran respondents not currently using cannabis to treat a medical condition

61%
Total respondents who do not currently know a veteran using cannabis to treat a medical condition

Would you want to have cannabis as a federally legal treatment?

Do you believe the federal government should legalize medical cannabis?

Do you support research into medical cannabis?

82% YES

83% YES

92% YES

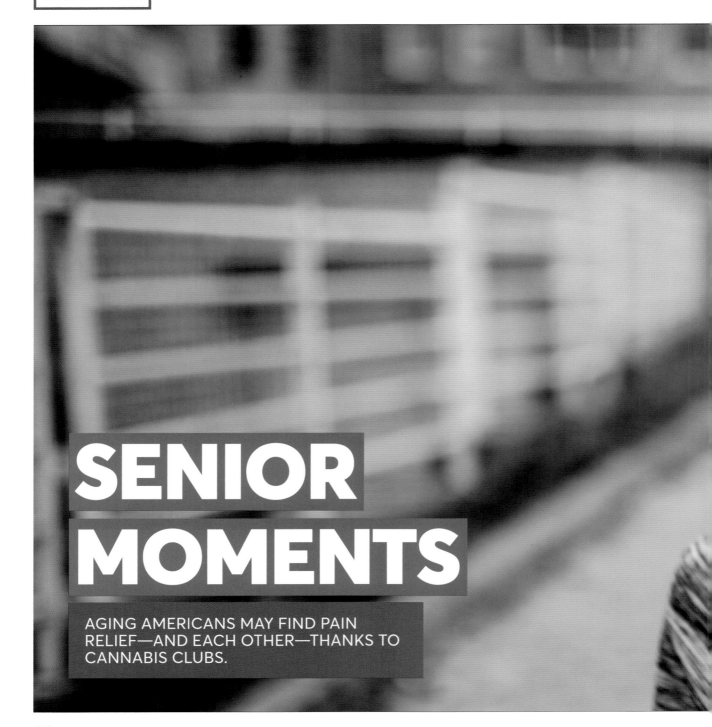

SENIOR MOMENTS

AGING AMERICANS MAY FIND PAIN RELIEF—AND EACH OTHER—THANKS TO CANNABIS CLUBS.

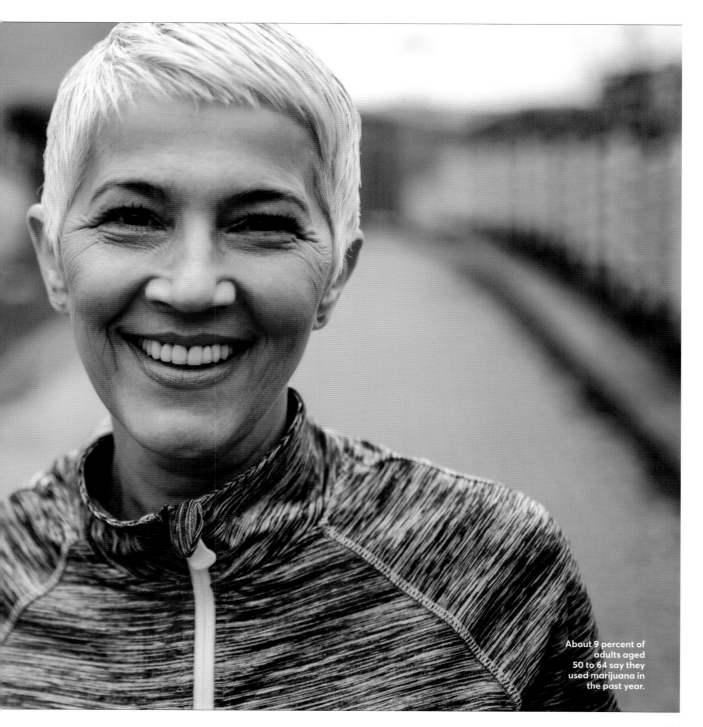

About 9 percent of adults aged 50 to 64 say they used marijuana in the past year.

Renee Lee is definitely no novice when it comes to cannabis. After all, she started smoking it back in 1968 after her sister turned her onto it—and subsequently growing up around musicians and other artistic types made it seem pretty normal. Still, it took the diagnosis of a brain tumor and obtaining her medical marijuana card in 2004 to introduce her to the full power of the plant. With the help of cannabis, she got off the "16 different pills they keep people on"—what she figures people are being given when they have cancer.

By 2011, Lee was living in Rossmoor, an upscale retirement community of about 10,000 that's located 25 miles east of San Francisco. That's when she noticed an ad in the local newspaper seeking fellow residents who might want to gather and hear more about marijuana, so Lee joined the 20 or so other folks who decided to attend. Now, eight years later, that little group has turned into Rossmoor's Medical Marijuana Education and Support Club, which gets about 200 people to show up for its meetings. And Lee has become its president.

"[Marijuana] has become a part of life here now," explains the 66-year-old therapist, who works with seniors who suffer from cognitive disabilities. "I can't go to the pool without people stopping me and having conversations about cannabis. It's become so much more normalized for everyone here now."

Since the club participants all came of age in a time when marijuana was demonized, Lee adds, they had plenty of fear about using it. Some worried that smoking might be bad for them. Others were concerned about getting high. But those concerns have been outweighed by the more real and pressing need to deal with the chronic pains of arthritis, insomnia, anxiety, depression and other health woes. Attending club meetings reassures them it's OK to consider marijuana as a valid alternative to the opioids that may be causing other problems.

Rossmoor residents aren't the only seniors who have rallied around cannabis in their community by starting a club. A few hours to the south, the Laguna Woods retirement community also had an organization that included hundreds of citizens. It even used its own grower to provide the marijuana used by residents. Changes in California laws no longer allow the club members to have their own collective, so the club disbanded and residents now travel together by bus to a nearby dispensary. Still, the fact that seniors are coming together to support each other when it comes to medical marijuana is a trend that's probably just beginning, given that cannabis use by U.S. adults 65 and over increased more than tenfold between 2007 and 2017.

SAFETY IN NUMBERS

"There is a massive aging population of baby boomers and their predecessors, and with aging comes arthritis, aches and pains and other health

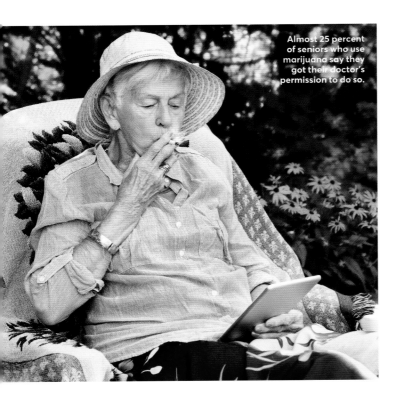

Almost 25 percent of seniors who use marijuana say they got their doctor's permission to do so.

CANNABIS COMES OF AGE

Just how effective is cannabis when it comes to treating senior citizens? A study conducted by the Dent Neurological Institute in Buffalo, New York, offers a few clues. Doctors looked at 204 people (average age: 81) who were enrolled in the New York State Medical Marijuana Program, and this is what they found:

69% of participants said they felt some degree of symptom relief from cannabis use.

18% saw an improvement with sleeping difficulties.

10% said that their anxiety problems got better.

34% said they experienced side effects from using cannabis.

13% of patients reported they'd experienced sleepiness as the most common side effect.

49% said they experienced relief from chronic pain.

15% reported improvement with neuropathy issues.

32% reported that they were able to reduce their opioid use.

21% experienced side effects, after an adjustment in their dosage.

7% had major side effects issues with balance and gastrointestinal issues.

problems," says Katie Stem, CEO of Peak Extracts, a leading cannabis company that specializes in the sort of CBD treatments popular with seniors. "The over-65 demographic is going to continue to pursue cannabis in greater numbers. Meanwhile, seniors tend to rely on the advice of community members and health providers before trying a new medication, so cannabis clubs, or talks organized within communities and nursing homes, are invaluable."

Lee's club has met regularly for several years, so members could hear speakers offering advice on everything from medical-marijuana recommendations to what delivery services can get medicine to residents. Her group has become so popular, she's actually starting a new one she says will be "more of a social club, where people can actually talk to each other" on a more one-to-one basis about what they're using and how it's working. "People can be fearful of standing up in large groups to ask questions and to talk," she explains. "They want to ask each other basic questions, like 'How do you read a label?' That is the core of what we're hoping to do: help people get over the fear of everything they've been taught about cannabis. When you're around friends who've used it, it's easier to try."

CBD IS THE CAT'S MEOW

CANNABIDIOL ISN'T JUST FOR PEOPLE. IT MAY BE PERFECT FOR PETS, TOO.

When Elizabeth Vernon discovered the healing effects of cannabis after a horrific car accident, she decided to treat some of the animals on her Northern New Jersey farm with the plant as well.

There's Delilah the duck, who was plagued with seizures. Billie Holiday, the chicken, who suffered from upper respiratory infections. And of course Sativa and Indica, two baby flying squirrels Vernon recently rescued. She says CBD cured the duck and chicken. As for the squirrels? "They have always been healthy. But I believe any animal—one as small as a mouse to one as big as an elephant—can benefit from CBD."

While Sativa and Indica may be the only flying squirrels ever to receive a daily dose of cannabis, Vernon is hardly alone in her beliefs. A recent survey found that 39 percent of dog owners and 34 percent of cat owners are in favor of treating pets with CBD supplements.

"It's hard to recall anything making more of a splash in both human and pet supplements than CBD," says David Sprinkle, research director for Packaged Facts, a market-research firm that conducted the survey.

As a groomer and trainer for 15 years, as well as a pet owner himself, Jeremy Feldman knew all too well about ailments that plague pets—anxiety, arthritis and joint pain. He also knew that common treatments, which often involved steroids, could prove more devastating than the ailments themselves. "I saw tons of health and behavior problems develop from these treatments—and I believed that there had to be some way for pet owners to deal with these issues that didn't involve dangerous solutions and expensive vet visits."

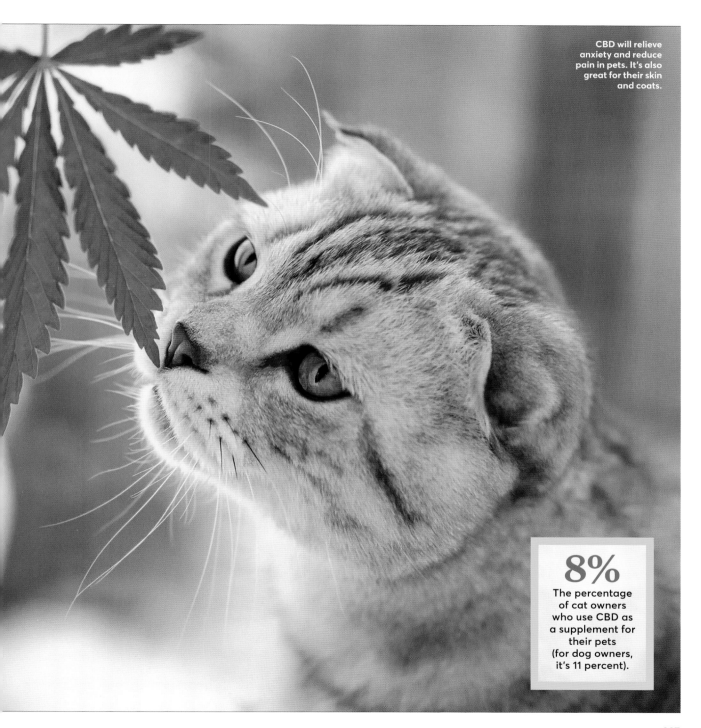

CBD will relieve anxiety and reduce pain in pets. It's also great for their skin and coats.

8%
The percentage of cat owners who use CBD as a supplement for their pets (for dog owners, it's 11 percent).

That's why he started Pet-Ness, a line of all-natural CBD pet treats, to support animal health. He's not alone. A multitude of CBD pet products—capsules, salves, tinctures and chew treats—have burst onto the market in the past few years. That's prompted experts to warn pet owners to proceed with caution if and when they decide to seek any of these items to treat their four-legged friends.

"It's the Wild West out there," says Elizabeth Mironchik-Frankenberg, DVM, a veterinarian and founder of Veterinary Cannabis Consultants, a CBD resource for veterinarians and consumers. "Everyone is trying to jump on the bandwagon to make money. There's confusion and misinformation about pet CBD. The good news is that since there's so much competition, there's no reason to settle for an inferior product."

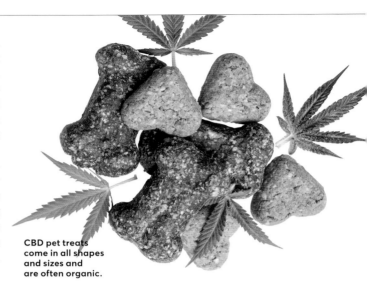

CBD pet treats come in all shapes and sizes and are often organic.

KENNEL CLUB STUDIES CBD

Since California is the only state that allows veterinarians to discuss cannabis with clients, consumers often don't know where to turn for advice. Adding to the confusion, producers of cannabis-infused edibles, tinctures and treats are limited in how they may advertise the products' benefits. Consumers have to be careful of wording. If a product is labeled "hemp-infused" or "hemp-based," it doesn't necessarily mean there is an appropriate level of CBD present. Also, since pet CBD is not FDA approved, the products don't undergo the same quality-control measures as medications for humans do.

As with CBD products for people, there isn't much research on the efficacy of CBD pet products. But this is beginning to change. A 2018 study at Cornell University's College of Veterinary Medicine concluded that 80 percent of the dogs in the study who took CBD oil for osteoarthritis showed "significant improvement in pain levels and quality of life" without discernible side effects. In 2017, the American Kennel Club Canine Health Foundation forked over $2 million for clinical trials to examine the use of CBD for drug-resistant epilepsy in dogs.

"CBD is remarkable for pets," says Feldman. "As more people understand its beneficial effects, there will be a lot more healthier and happier dogs and cats." Not to mention flying squirrels.

Pot Pet Tip

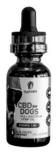

Be careful with dosages. Pets are much smaller than humans, and a too-high dose could result in oversedation.

Vetting CBD: Advice From an Expert

Figuring out the best CBD product and delivery method for your pet can be a daunting task, says Elizabeth Mironchik-Frankenberg, DVM. Here are some of her favorite tips:

1 Only California has passed legislation that authorizes vets to discuss cannabis with their clients. As a result, many vets don't know much about CBD. "As a pet owner, you have to be proactive. Don't expect vets to bring this up with you," Mironchik-Frankenberg says.

2 With so many products of varying quality on the market, pet owners need to do their due diligence. "You have to ask questions and do your research," she notes.

3 Look for the lab results, as well as the product's Certificate of Analysis. This will help ensure that the products have been formulated responsibly, are free of contaminants and contain the ingredients the product labels list. This information should be

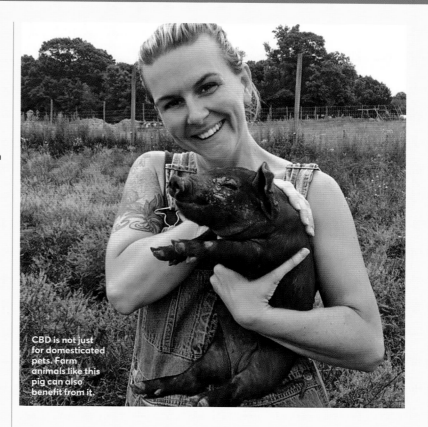

CBD is not just for domesticated pets. Farm animals like this pig can also benefit from it.

available on company websites. If not, email or call the company's customer service number and have them email the results to you. If they don't disclose this information, that's a major red flag, Mironchik-Frankenberg says.

4 Don't assume *your* CBD is OK for your pet. "There are ingredients that are perfectly

fine for humans, but toxic for pets," she explains.

5 Tinctures have recommended dosages based on your pet's size, but it can be hard to tell how much CBD a product contains. As with humans, it's best to start low and gradually increase the dosage based on your pet's needs in order to avoid overdosing.

HANDLE WITH CARE

MEDICAL-MARIJUANA PATIENTS ARE FINDING NEW ALLIES IN THEIR QUEST TO GET HEALTHY: CANNABIS CAREGIVERS.

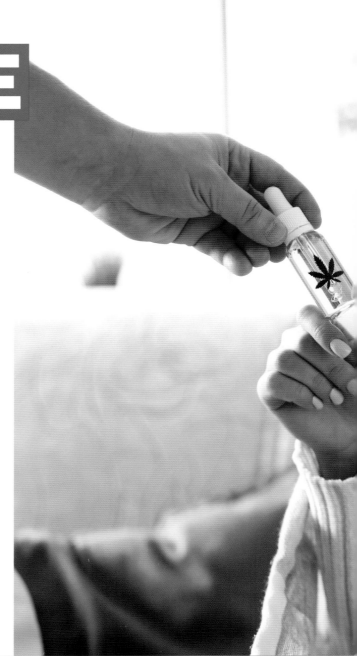

There's something very...clinical...about the phrase "cannabis caregiver." The "cannabis" part may seem cutting edge, but "caregiver" comes across as much more like something from traditional medicine. No matter how their title sounds, though, cannabis caregivers are rapidly becoming a very important part of the medical-marijuana world. Caregivers can help with procuring meds for those who are unable—whether due to age or infirmity—to buy or grow it for themselves. We spoke with Colorado-based cannabis

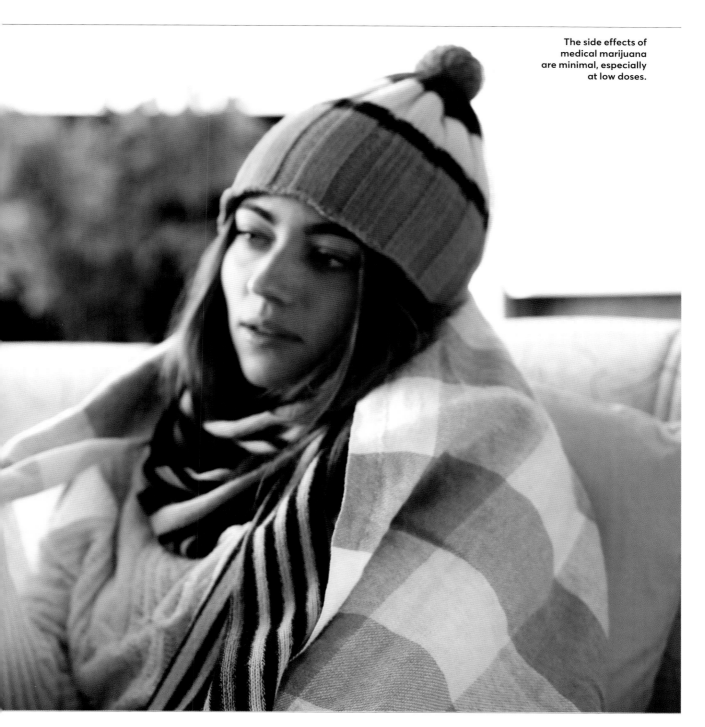

The side effects of medical marijuana are minimal, especially at low doses.

entrepreneur Karen Getchell, who creates courses for the online school Cannabis Training University (and is helping them develop a caregiver curriculum), to learn exactly what the job entails and how caregivers can help patients.

What exactly is a cannabis caregiver?

The cannabis caregiver is someone who helps a patient obtain medical cannabis, when the patient is not able to do that for himself or herself. Basically, if a patient is allowed to possess or cultivate a certain amount, the caregiver is also allowed to possess or cultivate that amount, in general. For instance, in many states, caregivers are required for minor patients. Usually, then, the caregiver is the parent or guardian.

Since cannabis laws vary from state to state, is the same true for regulations dealing with cannabis caregivers?

Every state has different rules. In some states, the patient has to designate a caregiver. But the caregiver will usually also have to go through an application process themselves and pay a fee. In some states, a caregiver has to be a certain age. In some states, the caregiver can't have any felony or drug convictions. So they have qualifications on their own. Sometimes they have to be related to the patient.

For instance, I can tell you the basic requirements in Colorado: The caregiver has to be at least 18 years old and a resident of Colorado. They cannot be the patient's physician. They cannot be a patient themselves, and they cannot be a licensed medical-cannabis business. Colorado's state program has four different types of caregivers: parents of a minor child; advising caregivers who provide advice on the medical use of cannabis; transporting caregivers, who basically pick up the cannabis and transport it to patients who are homebound; and cultivating caregivers, who grow cannabis for the patients. Only those who transport and cultivate cannabis are required to register with Colorado. And they can have up to five patients at once.

What are some of the common conditions that people using cannabis caregivers and medical marijuana suffer from?

It seems to me that the primary reason people get medical-cannabis cards is chronic pain. I think there are fewer people with epilepsy and cancer. PTSD is another big one.

What diseases or conditions lead people to seek out cannabis caregivers?

Each state has different qualifying conditions [for using medical marijuana]. Some states–like New York–are pretty rigid. There are only a few conditions. Other states, like Oklahoma, don't even have any qualifying conditions.

Is this a paid position?

In most cases, money is not exchanged–although patients are allowed, in some cases, to provide money to contribute to the cultivation of cannabis, for example.

Is there any medical licensing component to it, where people have to be certified to act as a caregiver, similar to how a pharmacist would be certified to dispense other drugs?

It's really more about acting as the patient in a purchasing, transporting and cultivating capacity when the patient can't do that themselves.

Once cannabis is legal in a state, is there still a call for cannabis caregivers?

Yes; for instance, sometimes it is about how far away you are from the nearest dispensary. You know, it might seem weird that somebody couldn't get in the car and go and get their medicine from a dispensary that is located right down the street. But in some states, the nearest dispensary might be 100 miles away. And the medical program will generally increase the limit of the amount of cannabis somebody is allowed to have in their possession.

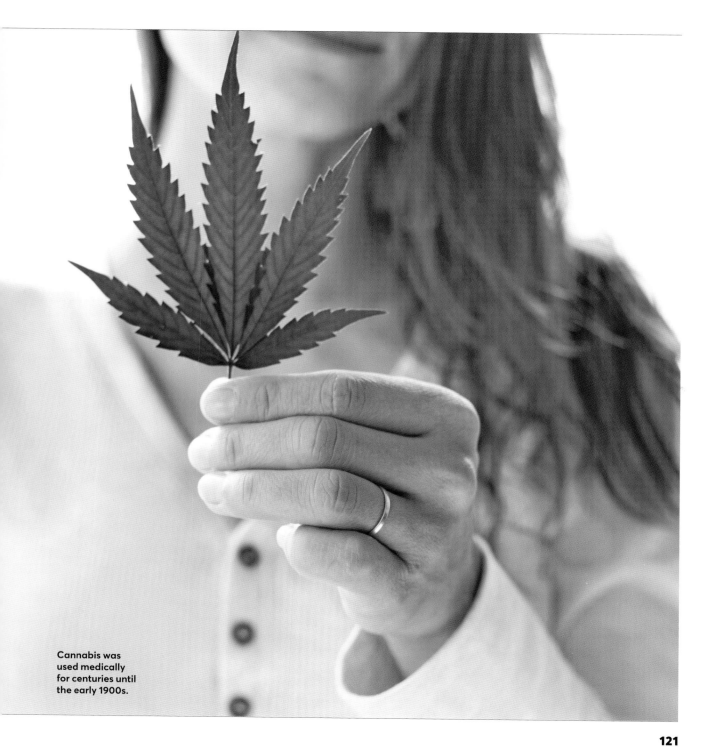

Cannabis was
used medically
for centuries until
the early 1900s.

IT'S ONLY NATURAL

HOLISTIC HEALERS ARE CONNECTING WITH CANNABIS TO ENHANCE THEIR THERAPIES.

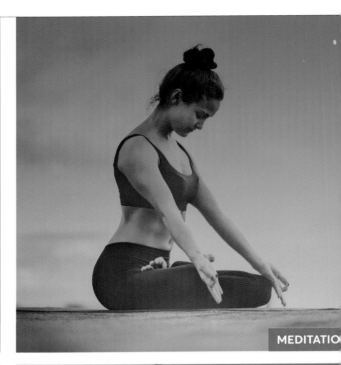

MEDITATIO

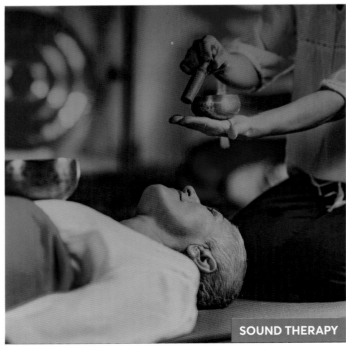

SOUND THERAPY

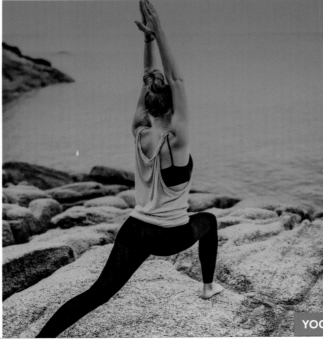

YO

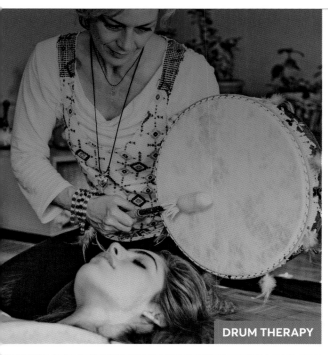

DRUM THERAPY

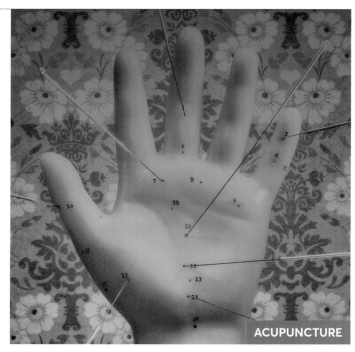

ACUPUNCTURE

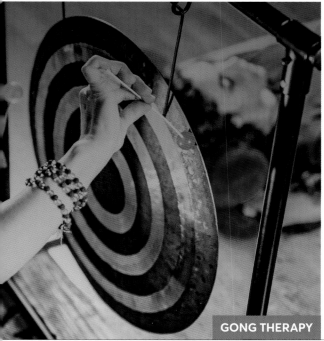

GONG THERAPY

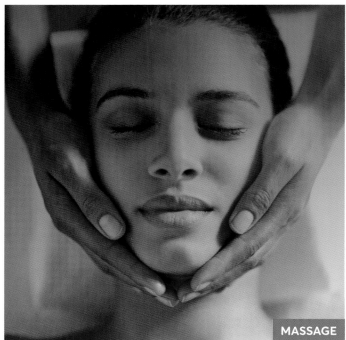

MASSAGE

There's no doubt that part of the growing appeal of medical marijuana is the fact that it is health care that comes from the ground and not from any laboratory. It's as natural as a treatment can get. Or, at least it was, until recently. These days, healers have started blending the power of cannabis with a variety of holistic health regimens to re-establish the body's balance and jump-start wellness in as pure a way as possible. Here are some therapies that combine weed and new-age remedies.

ON PLANTS AND NEEDLES

Chinese healers have used acupuncture, along with cannabis, for thousands of years. But it was only after the human endocannabinoid system (ECS) was discovered a couple of decades ago that researchers realized both weed and needles can stimulate the ECS to promote homeostasis in the body, allowing for optimal healing. However, weed and needles tend to act in very different ways. Acupuncture uses needles that are inserted just below the skin at specific points along the body, known as meridians, in order to unblock the energy flow and stimulate the ECS. Blocked energy, healers say, can potentially cause body aches, imbalance and disease. Meanwhile, with cannabis, the phytocannabinoids within the plant interact with the ECS through its receptors.

Although they get to the ECS in different ways, acupuncture needles and marijuana can work together to soothe inflammation and pain. Hayley Jackson, a licensed acupuncturist at San Francisco's Truspine clinic, is very familiar with this joint treatment. For instance, she likes to incorporate CBD salve with traditional acupuncture to treat sore muscles, anxiety and insomnia. "Many patients get faster and longer-lasting results when I combine acupuncture and cannabis," says Jackson, adding that the CBD salve is especially useful after dry needling to relieve soreness.

THE SOUND (BATH) AND THE GREEN

One of the latest trends in holistic healing is the sound bath, a form of therapy that uses music and rhythm to soothe anxiety and stress, allowing the body to rest and heal, according to Seth Misterka, a meditation teacher and member of the group Dynasty Electrik. "It's like a concert experience, except you lie down and have the music wash over you," he explains.

Misterka and his partner, Jenny Deveau, provide these sound baths to help their clients counter the effects of all of life's stresses. The duo incorporates a variety of very different sounds into its treatments– including singing bowls, gongs, chimes, drums and native American flutes. Each of these instruments provides a different benefit. Misterka plays the bowls above the client's body to identify where there is an imbalance. "As a sound healer, I seek to tune people's nervous systems. The bowls correspond to chakra centers associated with specific areas of the body," he explains. The sound bath harmonizes the discordant frequency to promote healing.

He and Deveau like to use cannabis at the start of their sound sessions to deepen the experience for clients. "It becomes an inner visual experience," Misterka says. "You move into your own body and your own mind."

The Dynasty Electrik duo is convinced that cannabis is an appropriate healing tool, provided it is used properly and there's some thought behind the process. "People come to us to deal with emotional trauma or specific pain," says Deveau. "Sound healing and cannabis move the body back into balance and aid in well-being."

YOGA GOES GANJA

A decade ago, San Francisco-based yoga instructor Dee Dussault decided it was time to create the first public, cannabis-enhanced yoga classes after realizing that the fulfilled feeling she got from marijuana might perfectly complement the glorious glow she experienced in her yoga practice. Now, she's the founder of the Ganja Yoga practice and author of the book *Ganja Yoga*, regularly witnessing how weed paired with yoga can ease pain and inflammation in her students.

"[Cannabis] lets people feel more connected to their bodies, which creates more mindfulness and creativity in a [yoga] practice," Dussault explains.

Each class begins with her students sampling cannabis prior to getting out on their mats for an hour of yoga and meditation. They are allowed to take weed breaks during their session and linger for a while afterward to sober up. Dussault designs her classes for all body types and all ages and has seen that cannabis helps even the most nervous of newbies to shake off their anxiety about striking a yoga pose.

Says Dussault, "Yoga has over 75 health benefits and, like cannabis, one of yoga's main benefits is that it helps people relax. The two work symbiotically to fight both inflammation and anxiety."

■ MARIJUANA MASSAGES

As it turns out, marijuana can rub you the right way. At least that's the motivating factor behind Primal Therapeutics, a mobile cannabis-massage provider in the Denver area. The company offers massages—using a variety of cannabis-infused oils, along with information about the healing power of marijuana—by licensed massage therapists. Founded five years ago by Jordan Person, a nurse and massage therapist herself, Primal Therapeutics uses whole-plant—infused lotions to activate ECS receptors that exist on the surface of the skin.

While there's no concrete scientific proof as to what medicinal benefits cannabis-infused massages provide, Person started tracking clients' post-massage improvements in a spreadsheet. This led her to conclude using cannabis with massage can amplify the therapeutic benefits from the massage, soothing pain and areas of discomfort. In fact, the combo has left some clients so relaxed, they didn't even need to apply ice after their sessions to relieve discomfort following deep-tissue massages.

"The topical cannabis lotions used during the massage also worked as an anti-inflammatory," concludes Person.

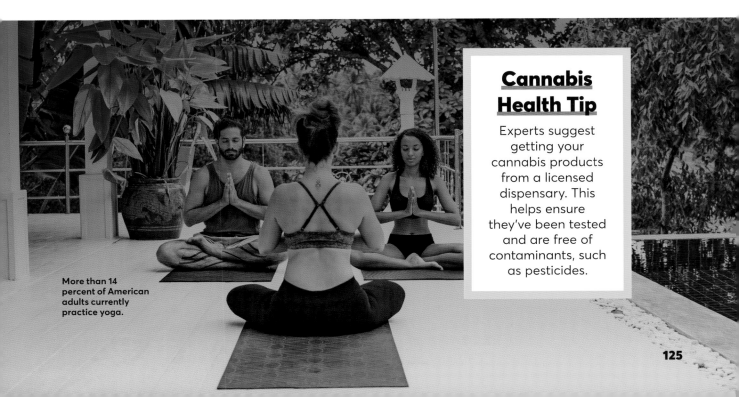

More than 14 percent of American adults currently practice yoga.

Cannabis Health Tip

Experts suggest getting your cannabis products from a licensed dispensary. This helps ensure they've been tested and are free of contaminants, such as pesticides.

POT CROCK?

MARIJUANA HAS INSPIRED MANY MYTHS. HERE'S THE LOWDOWN ON WHAT'S FACT AND WHAT'S FICTION.

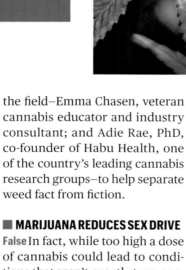

Sit too close to the TV, and you'll ruin your eyesight. Go swimming less than an hour after eating, and you'll cramp up. Make a weird face, and it'll stick like that. Whether they were meant to terrify us or soothe us, these urban legends and many more have long been a part of our lives. So it should come as no surprise that a mythology has also sprung up around cannabis. So many questionable myths have hung around for so long, it's hard to know what's true and what are remnants from the *Reefer Madness* era. To clear things up, we asked two experts in

the field–Emma Chasen, veteran cannabis educator and industry consultant; and Adie Rae, PhD, co-founder of Habu Health, one of the country's leading cannabis research groups–to help separate weed fact from fiction.

■ MARIJUANA REDUCES SEX DRIVE

False In fact, while too high a dose of cannabis could lead to conditions that aren't exactly turn-ons, like drowsiness, anxiety and/or paranoia, the appropriate dose might actually improve your sex life. "For females with low libido, cannabis appears to be a viable therapy to enhance it," says Rae.

Chasen agrees that it can up your sex drive because marijuana "increases blood flow, and there are endocannabinoid receptors densely populated in our reproductive systems, increasing sensation and often diminishing pain."

■ MARIJUANA IS HIGHLY ADDICTIVE

Mostly False If you want to talk about substances that encourage addiction, Rae suggests discussing nicotine or alcohol instead, since they are the real offenders. Chasen does point out that to be technically addictive, a substance must produce measurable withdrawal

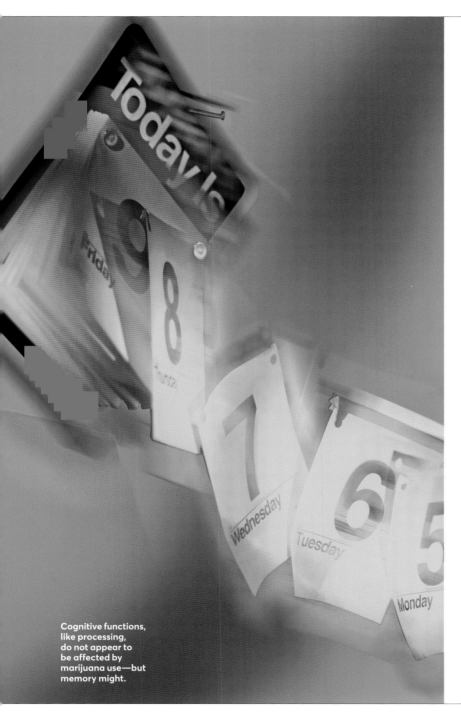

Cognitive functions, like processing, do not appear to be affected by marijuana use—but memory might.

and tolerance–which cannabis does. "Withdrawal symptoms may leave you grumpy, in some pain and not able to sleep, but they definitely won't kill you. And while tolerance can be developed to the psychoactivity of THC, tolerance to the benefits of THC cannot. Therefore, THC can be considered addictive, but it's not an addiction that will likely ruin your life."

■ MARIJUANA STAYS IN YOUR SYSTEM FOR 30 DAYS

True Cannabinoids are lipids, which are the same thing that your fat tissue is made of. This means that when you ingest cannabis, its molecules get stored in your body's fat tissue. Rae says that those who use cannabis more than twice a week can expect to have detectable levels of it in their urine for up to 30 days, although there is a lot of variability, depending upon a person's body metabolism and physiology.

■ MARIJUANA CAUSES SHORT-TERM MEMORY LOSS

Somewhat True According to Rae, "THC impairs some kinds of cognitive function but not others." However, she adds that THC's impact on memory formation is "largely dose-dependent." The effects of low doses of THC have not been measured. Chasen adds that while excessive THC "may lead to short-term memory loss," especially in young adults, there are compounds in cannabis (particularly one called pinene) that can offset this potential problem.

ALL CBD OILS ARE THE SAME

False With hemp-derived CBD products flooding the market, buyers need to be wary of what they're getting. "Craft hemp," as it's often called (a la "craft beer"), may be everywhere but according to Rae, it also has less than 0.3 percent THC. There's still a wide range of therapeutically valuable molecules in there even with virtually no THC. However, the highest-quality CBD oils feature what she says is a "full spectrum" of ingredients that come from organically grown cannabis and not "the fibrous industrial hemp that contains minimal beneficial ingredients."

YOU CAN OVERDOSE ON MEDICAL CANNABIS

True and False Technically, says Chasen, this is possible–if you define overdose as simply taking too much of a substance. "Operating with this definition, a lot of people overdose on cannabis and have anxious, paranoid experiences," she explains, adding that "you cannot lethally overdose on cannabis. There are no CB1 receptors in brain stem cardiorespiratory centers, which means cannabis cannot shut down essential functions, such as breathing and heartbeat. To date, there have been no reported deaths due to an overdose of cannabis."

MAJOR MEDICAL ORGANIZATIONS DON'T SUPPORT MEDICAL-MARIJUANA USE

True However, the reluctance of organizations like the American Medical Association to get onboard with cannabis has more to do with the fact that it is still federally prohibited, and there's next to no endocannabiology education in medical schools due to an inherent mistrust of the plant. "This is slowly evolving," explains Rae. "The AMA and other large medical societies have too much to lose in terms of federal credibility to amend their policies."

MARIJUANA CAUSES GYNECOMASTIA

False It's highly unlikely pot causes male breast development, but Rae admits there is "very sparse evidence" for this belief dating back at least to the 1960s. She cites a case report from the '70s and another from 2007 that found THC had effects on both male and female gonadal hormones. But she adds, "these are very complex interactions. Some individuals may be more at risk than others. It may also be dose-dependent, but no studies have been done." Chasen says that cannabis shouldn't be a direct cause of gynecomastia, which is a disorder caused by hormonal imbalance.

CBD CAN CURE ANYTHING

False Even cannabis's most passionate supporters admit CBD has its limits. "It's a compound

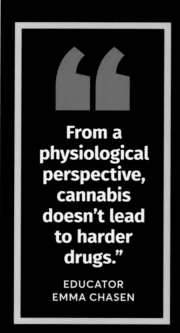

From a physiological perspective, cannabis doesn't lead to harder drugs."

EDUCATOR
EMMA CHASEN

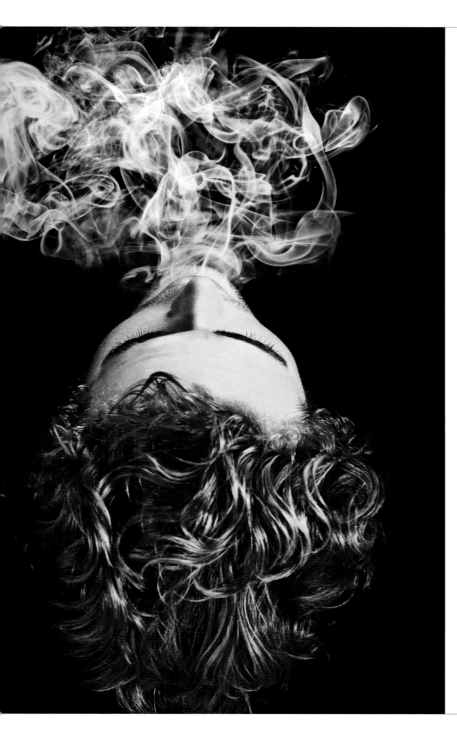

with large therapeutic potential," says Chasen. "However, to improve efficacy, it must be taken in a holistic context. CBD won't cure you of anything, and it may not even help you if you continue to sacrifice health and care in other areas of your life." Still, Rae adds, CBD does have a "very powerful placebo effect," which can be a "psychological tool for managing chronic disease. Allowing your brain to think that a substance is going to truly work is often more powerful than the substance itself."

■ MARIJUANA LEADS TO HARDER DRUGS

False Marijuana opponents have long called it a "gateway" drug, which may lead to the use of more addictive and potentially dangerous substances, but Chasen sees that more as a social trait of cannabis rather than a physical one. "From a social behavior examination, people who consume cannabis may have traditionally been more likely to consume other illicit substances," he says. "But from a physiological perspective, cannabis doesn't lead to harder drugs. It does not cause a change in the body that would make it more likely for people to seek out other, more dangerous substances." Likewise, Rae admits that while cannabis use is "correlated with the use of harder drugs, so are alcohol use and nicotine use. 'Correlation' and 'causation' are not the same."

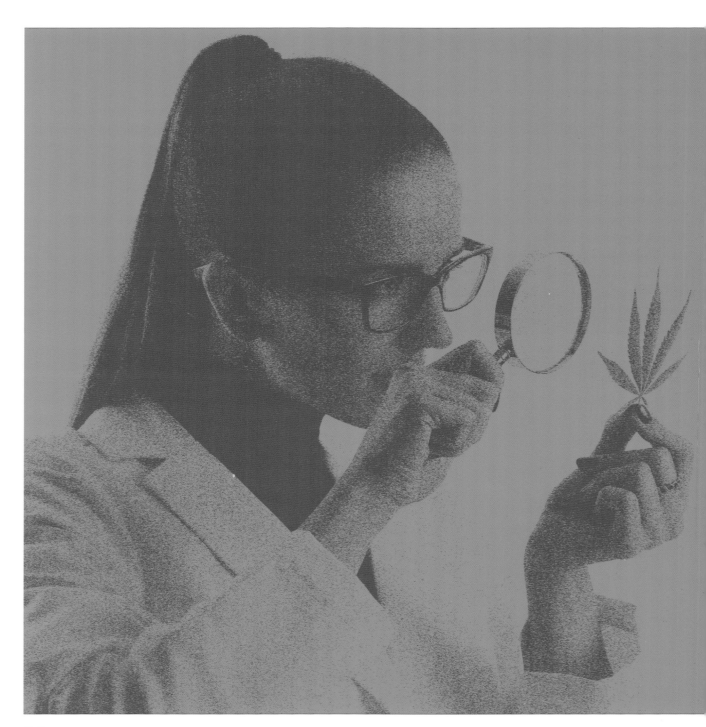

PART 3

CANNABIS CHAMPIONS

POT'S PATRON SAINT

FOR TOMMY CHONG, CANNABIS HAS BEEN A LAUGHING MATTER— AND A LIFESAVER.

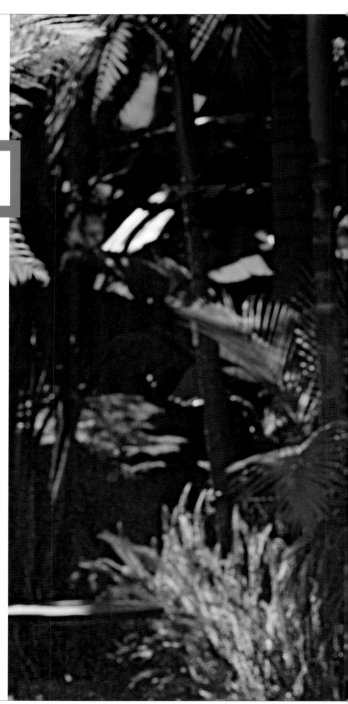

When you think of certain iconic historical figures, there are particular items associated with them that inevitably come to mind. Isaac Newton and his apple, for instance. Abe Lincoln and that hat. Michael Jackson and the glove. Likewise, when you think of Tommy Chong, it's virtually impossible to picture the veteran comedian without also seeing a cloud of smoke.

Throughout the 1970s and 1980s, along with his partner, Cheech Marin, Chong released nine comedy albums, including Big Bambu and the Grammy Award-winning Los Cochinos. The pair also made eight feature

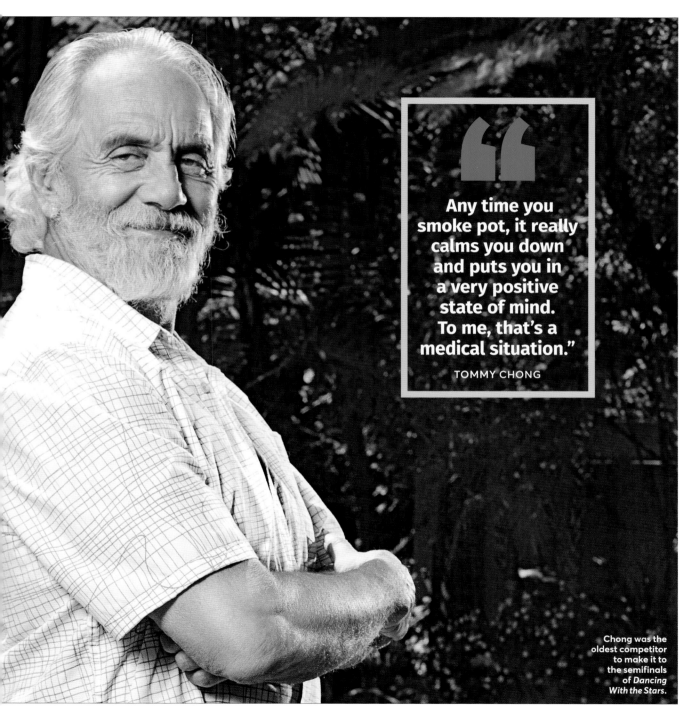

> ❝ Any time you smoke pot, it really calms you down and puts you in a very positive state of mind. To me, that's a medical situation. ❞
>
> TOMMY CHONG

Chong was the oldest competitor to make it to the semifinals of *Dancing With the Stars*.

films during that time, including Up In Smoke *and* Still Smokin'. *And the one thing that tied every project together? Marijuana.*

Cheech & Chong were the patron saints of pot, vocal advocates for the drug in a time when the country had declared war upon it and those who used it. Well, the times have certainly changed–but Tommy Chong hasn't. He continues to be a tireless proponent of marijuana but with one big difference: Now he's seen firsthand the medical benefits of cannabis.

In 2012, he battled stage I prostate cancer–and, after seeing it go into remission, was stricken in 2015 by colorectal cancer. True to form, he used marijuana to recover in both cases–and has now made pot his business, literally. Along with his son Paris, he started Chong's Choice, a line of cannabis products that includes everything from clothing to CBD oils. We spoke with Chong about his cancer bouts and how important marijuana has been in regaining his health.

The truth is I was always cautious when it came to smoking marijuana. When I was 16, I got turned on to bodybuilding, and when you're into that, you have to be careful what you put into your body. You have to stop drinking soft drinks. You can't eat hamburgers and junk food. I learned Arnold Schwarzenegger would spit out liquor but that at his peak in bodybuilding, the only thing he would do is smoke pot. The healthiest man on the planet wouldn't do anything else. So I knew from my earliest bodybuilding experiences that marijuana made you hungry for good food and made you more creative. I wasn't getting high to forget or to party or to rob a bank. I wasn't using pot for evil purposes.

◼ COMING TO TERMS WITH CANCER

When I started smoking marijuana, it was the evil drug that was going to make you get high and kill your parents. We all hid it from each other. I was in a band and didn't even know the piano player was smoking too. Plus, I was always a one-toker. I've never been a heavy smoker. I remember being given a joint and a

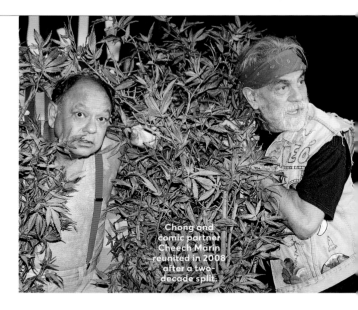

Chong and comic partner Cheech Marin reunited in 2008 after a two-decade split.

Lenny Bruce record at the same time, and the joint lasted me a month. That's a habit I continue to this day.

Still, back in the day when Cheech and I were together, we were considered horrible because we were supposedly promoting youth drug use. One time I did an interview and asked, 'What if we're right, and it turns out marijuana is actually good for you? What if that happens?' Cheech loved that and still quotes it. The strange thing is, that has actually come true.

I got to know this personally after I was diagnosed with prostate cancer, which doctors discovered because I was about to start doing testosterone shots. My son and I are both bodybuilders, and he'd told me I was at the age where testosterone gets low–so I should consider starting the shots. In order to do that, you have to get a complete physical checkup to make sure you don't have cancer, because growth hormones can promote cancer growth. So that's when I got the news: I had prostate cancer.

I went to a holistic doctor, and he put me on a strict diet. He said that it was a slow-moving cancer, and I'd probably die of something else before it got to me. So I tried the holistic approach–and that's when I started

SIX CELEBRITIES WHO SUPPORT MEDICAL MARIJUANA

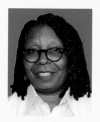

WHOOPI GOLDBERG

The comedian, actress and *View* host partnered with businesswoman Maya Elisabeth in 2016 to create the company Maya & Whoopi, which sells cannabis products aimed at relieving menstrual cramps.

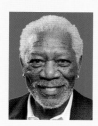

MORGAN FREEMAN

The Oscar-winning actor developed fibromyalgia pain in his arm following a near-fatal car crash in 2008. He has said in the past that "the only thing that offers any relief is marijuana."

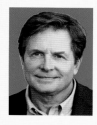

MICHAEL J. FOX

A victim of Parkinson's disease, the actor set up a foundation to help others suffering from it as well. And in 2017, that group lobbied Congress to consider marijuana as legal for relief from pain associated with Parkinson's.

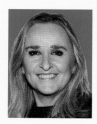

MELISSA ETHERIDGE

Stricken with breast cancer in 2004, the Grammy Award-winning musician credits marijuana with helping her beat the disease. In 2017, she launched Etheridge Farms, a line of cannabis-related products.

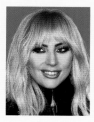

LADY GAGA

Overwhelmed by chronic pain from her fibromyalgia, the singer has reportedly relied on marijuana to help manage the agony.

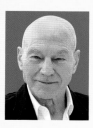

PATRICK STEWART

The *Star Trek* star revealed in 2017 that he uses cannabis ointments, sprays and edibles to help with debilitating arthritis.

reading about how marijuana worked [medically]. I started using marijuana suppositories and hemp oil. Then I got on *Dancing With the Stars,* and it was so hard on me physically. I could tell that I was experiencing the symptoms of rectal cancer, but I put off dealing with it until I finished the show. Then I was told that I had a tumor on my rectum.

■ THE ROCKY ROAD TO RECOVERY

I had smoked occasionally with my prostate cancer. However, to go into this heavy treatment for rectal cancer, I decided to go with straight medicine to treat it. My son Paris was with me when a woman approached me with the theory that chemo and radiation will kill you, and I should get off them and do marijuana instead. Paris had been with me throughout my whole journey. He had talked to the cancer doctors, so he asked her, "What's your backup on this?" She couldn't answer. It was all just rumors. I had a choice. I could have taken the Farrah Fawcett approach. She tried holistic stuff like coffee enemas, but the cancer killed her. What happens if you treat using other things without radiation...it's like throwing gasoline on the fire.

I got off marijuana for the surgery and the chemo. I did the pills and radiation and never had the urge to do marijuana until after that was done. Then I used it to get off the opioids I'd been given, like OxyContin. I kicked those drugs with no problem. And I honestly don't think I'd be alive today if I hadn't used marijuana. After the operation, I had no appetite and was addicted to the opioids I was given. When you're addicted to something, you don't realize you're addicted. All you know is you have a date, you have to get there and you have to put this sh-t in your veins. Marijuana

cleared my mind and gave me not only an appetite but also creative urges I hadn't had for a while.

One of the most dangerous things that happens when you get deathly ill, like I was, is that you lose your appetite—and within days, all your organs are in danger of starvation. When you're fighting disease, though, you need all the good stuff in your body that you can get. Marijuana not only gives you the good state of mind that you need, it brings back your appetite.

My health is excellent now. I try to work out three or four times a week. Even when I was sick, I never stopped working out. The day after my operation, I was doing planks. I've found the biggest problem as you get old is that we sit down too much; it throws the body out of whack. The secret of life is to keep moving.

What you'll find is that when people smoke marijuana, they get into an altered state—and regardless of what your medical condition is, it seems to be positive in every way, except for schizophrenia. I think it doesn't work for that, but I don't have any statistics. With everything else, any time you smoke pot, it really calms you down and puts you in a very positive state of mind. To me, that's a medical situation. It changes your mood, your attitude, your entire outlook. And that's what medicine is supposed to do.

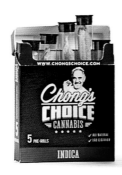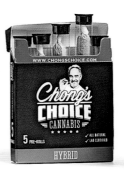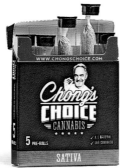

Chong's Choice products are available in several states.

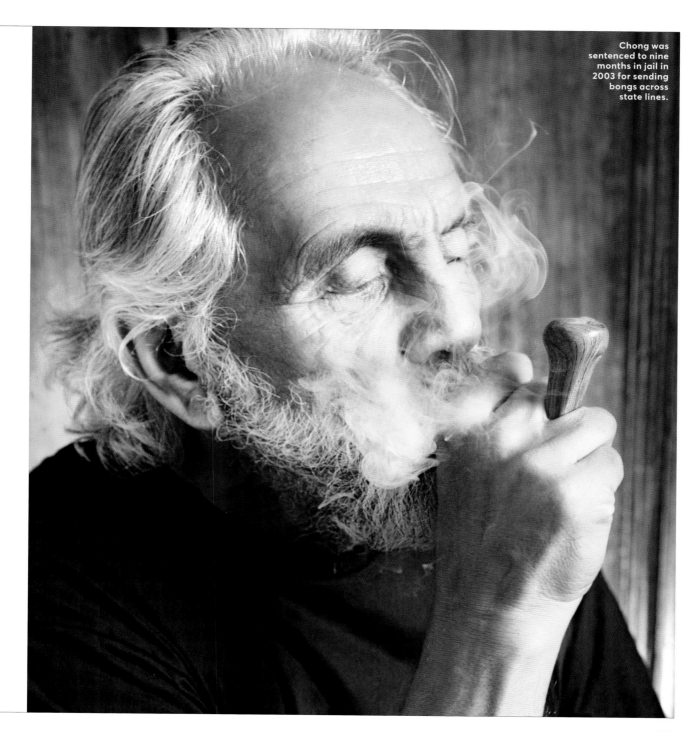

Chong was sentenced to nine months in jail in 2003 for sending bongs across state lines.

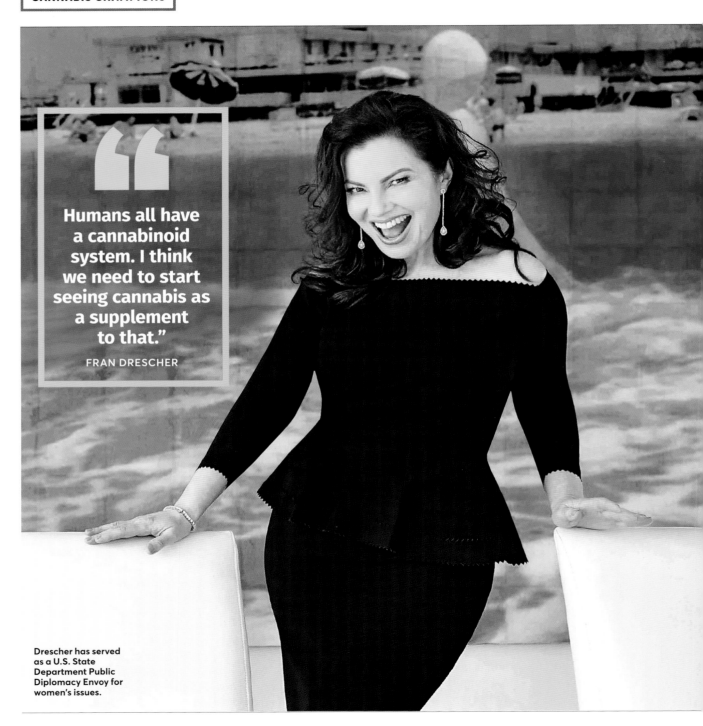

> "Humans all have a cannabinoid system. I think we need to start seeing cannabis as a supplement to that."
>
> FRAN DRESCHER

Drescher has served as a U.S. State Department Public Diplomacy Envoy for women's issues.

A TRUE BELIEVER

THE *NANNY* STAR FRAN DRESCHER IS FAMOUSLY FUNNY, BUT THESE DAYS SHE'S GETTING SERIOUS ABOUT MEDICAL CANNABIS.

Fran Drescher has always had a knack for looking right into the face of serious challenges over the years. For instance, there was the difficulty of making her way in Hollywood as an unknown actor. And the horror of being diagnosed with uterine cancer, having a radical hysterectomy and discovering her appendix had unexpectedly been removed during surgery. Then, there was coping with the news that her father was suffering from Parkinson's disease.

However, it was when she was looking into his face that she saw something truly transformative. To deal with the symptoms of his illness, he'd tried medical cannabis—and there was no hiding the difference it made.

"Suddenly, there was more expression in his face," recalls the 61-year-old actor and former star of the hit '90s CBS sitcom *The Nanny*. "Yes, he still had Parkinson's, but cannabis was helping him connect with his body more. His face got more animated. You could see it in his eyes. He was back to being himself. It was very helpful with his ability to animate and feel grounded in his body."

She was already a believer in the powers of the plant, but this experience with her dad reaffirmed her desire to take that interest to the next level. These days, while she continues to work as an actor and an author—she's written two *New York Times* best-sellers, *Enter Whining* and *Cancer Schmancer*—Drescher has also become a major proponent of medical-marijuana use. That advocacy includes her annual Master Class Health Summit in Los Angeles, where attendees can get wellness advice from a variety of leading physicians, including some with an expertise in healing through CBD and THC.

Drescher took some time to share details about her journey from comedy star to cannabis supporter, and how she came to view the plant as a power for good.

You're certainly not alone in your support of medical cannabis use these days. A majority of states now have some sort of formal program for it. Are you surprised at all about how quickly it's becoming an accepted form of treatment?

I absolutely expected this to happen. It wasn't like people weren't using it before and suddenly they are. This was a recreational street drug, but tons of people were using it. The fact that it's still a Schedule 1 drug is truly outrageous, but sometimes you have to have a grassroots movement like we're seeing in order to change things.

Was there any particular moment in your life where the potential healing powers of cannabis really hit home for you?

I think it was when I started to see how it helped with my own chronic issues, like inflammation and stress levels. It was after I went to Vienna to get a lifetime achievement award and threw my back out before going to the event. A doctor came to help get me off the floor, and I showed her that my hands were all swollen. She said I had a histamine issue, a problem metabolizing it. I went to all kinds of doctors and... long story short...they put me on a no-histamine diet for a month, and if the symptoms went away, they'd know what my problem was. It's just not possible to manage [histamine intake] 24 hours a day because there's a lot of toxic environments out there, and when

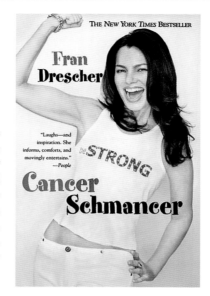

In her 2002 book *Cancer Schmancer*, Drescher chronicled her recovery from uterine cancer.

you're around them, the body will start to produce [histamines]. So what I found by using cannabis at that time was that it really seemed to help with the inflammation. And that was when I really started to get more engaged in using it again.

Was it strange to think that this illicit thing you used to use as a teenager was now something that made you feel better at this stage of your life?

I had to wrap my mind around the idea that using [cannabis] is like taking a vitamin. You have to think of it that way. You have to get comfortable with the fact that we're dealing with something that's a

more natural, earthy product, and there will be more variables [than with prescription medications]. It's detaching ourselves from thinking the best way to feel better is to take a pill at 11 in the morning, another in the afternoon and another before bed. And if it doesn't work for you, at least you gave it a shot. There's really no downside to trying it. You're not going to overdose; you're not going to die; you're not going to get lung cancer. And usually, in varying degrees, it helps people. This is a very useful plant that has made multiple contributions to the modern world, and we should treat it right, from seed to user.

What advice do you have for people who are still new to medical marijuana and unsure about it all?

Start very small. Titrate and keep water and food by your side as you find what's right for you. And journal. Keep a record of what you're doing that you can go back and check. That's very important.

Were you much of a user when you were younger, particularly as you recovered from your cancer surgery?

I was a social user prior to getting sick but I didn't indulge immediately after surgery. It was a little bit hard to handle at that time. When I tried to smoke, I felt too high. However, then I ended up going back to it to control my inflammation, and it's been helpful with that since then.

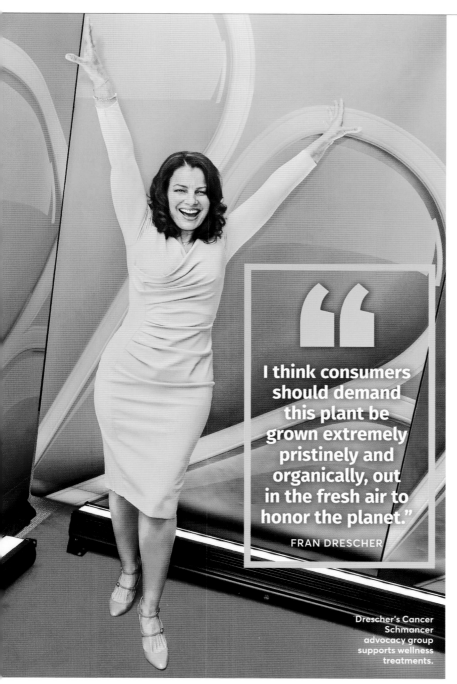

> **I think consumers should demand this plant be grown extremely pristinely and organically, out in the fresh air to honor the planet."**
>
> FRAN DRESCHER

Drescher's Cancer Schmancer advocacy group supports wellness treatments.

Do you have a preferred way of using cannabis?

I'm still old-school. I like to smoke, usually with a pipe or organic paper. It works faster, and it's also over quicker, so I feel like I can control it better. Having said that, I know a lot of people who love their edibles because it helps them sleep at night. I'm not really a fan of the vape pen, but maybe I just haven't found what gives me a nice feeling yet. I also have nothing against using something with THC in it. In fact, that's the stuff that works on the brain. My dad absolutely has to have his THC. I don't think there's anything wrong with including it in whatever you choose to use.

You've spoken at cannabis conferences in the past and you host an annual Master Class Health Summit. What should people expect to see theres?

We have panels where people can hear compelling stories from those who have been helped [by cannabis]. There are people who write cookbooks about how you can put it in your food. We're all about self-empowerment. You are the medical consumer. You know what you need. Partner with your doctor, explain what you suspect is the problem and don't become infantile with him or her. It's important to empower and engage ourselves in this way and that absolutely includes seeing cannabis as a first option and not a last one.

CANNABIS CONVERT

AFTER YEARS AS A SKEPTIC, CNN'S DR. SANJAY GUPTA HAS BECOME A SUPPORTER OF MEDICAL MARIJUANA.

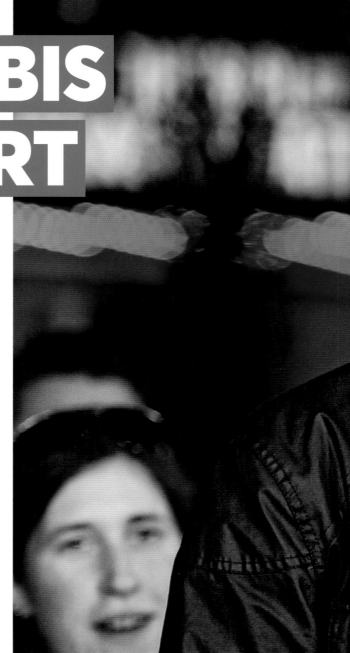

There was a time, not that long ago, when Sanjay Gupta, MD, was certain he knew the evil truth about marijuana. In a 2009 essay for *Time* magazine, the neurosurgeon and CNN commentator couldn't have been any clearer in his assessment of medical cannabis, writing, "I'm here to tell you, as a doctor, that despite all the talk about the medical benefits of marijuana, smoking the stuff is not going to do your health any good."

The way he saw it, there was very little reliable scientific evidence to support the belief in cannabis as a cure-all. "Most of the papers published on the topic weren't particularly impressive to me," he now recalls. "They weren't talking about the benefits of medical marijuana."

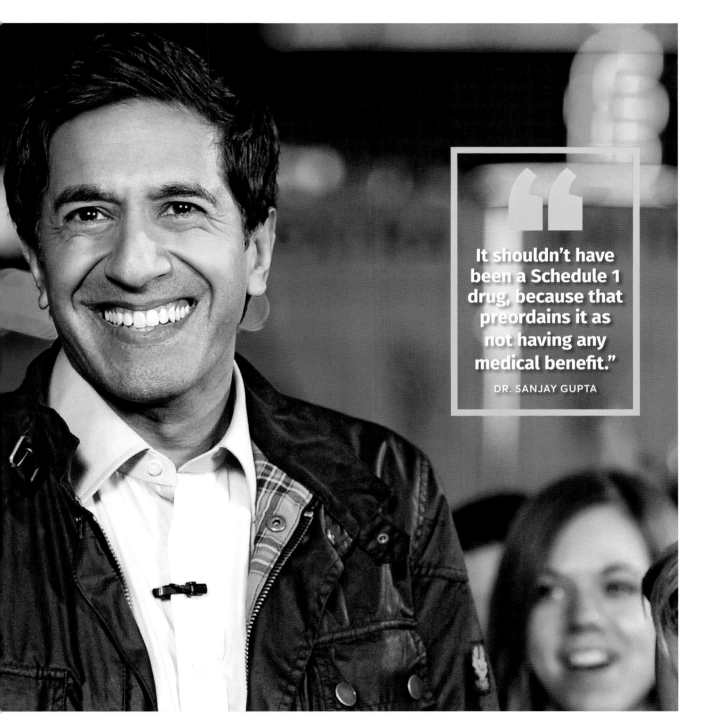

> **It shouldn't have been a Schedule 1 drug, because that preordains it as not having any medical benefit."**
>
> DR. SANJAY GUPTA

It's been more than 10 years and five CNN *Weed* documentaries since that essay, however— and these days, nobody is a bigger believer in the potential power of medical marijuana than Dr. Gupta. We talked with him about the reasons for this turnaround, the best uses for cannabis and where the research into medical marijuana goes from here.

Was there a particular moment when your opinions about the use of medicinal marijuana changed?
Actually, there were a couple of moments that turned it around for me. The first was meeting Charlotte Figi for our first *Weed* documentary. She was a young girl who had refractory epilepsy that was unresponsive to six or seven generations of epilepsy drugs. She was constantly having seizures, and she was never able to be out of her parents' sight. By age 3, she was having 300 a week. Some treatments had even put her into cardiac arrest. When you have something like that, it affects everyone in your world a lot. Then, when she started using CBD oil, she had a significant improvement. In fact, Charlotte's Web [a cannabis extract used to control seizures] was named after her. As a doctor and someone who has written a lot of papers on a lot of subjects, I realize you have to be supercareful relying on anecdotal stories for information. But Charlotte's story was very gripping.

Can you describe the other moment when your thinking changed?
It came while researching the CNN films. I approached them the way I approach everything I do, but researching medical marijuana required more digging. There were many papers written about medical marijuana that were available in 2010, and I could pie-chart them into a hypothesis showing that they were looking more for the harm than the benefits. That was the approach that was getting the research funding—so when you'd apply for a grant, if you said you wanted to look at the

harm rather than the benefits, you'd have more luck. It's a little nuanced, but it was almost like the system was rigged a bit.

Marijuana has been demonized for much of the past century even though, historically, it's been known to help a wide variety of medical maladies. Why do you think that is?
I know it was on the drug formulary [a list of prescription drugs that doctors have approved for use] until the early 1940s. At the time, there was something going on culturally, such as the Hearst-funded propaganda films that portrayed marijuana use in a negative light. Even when it became a Schedule 1 substance in the '70s, those who were writing about marijuana said there wasn't enough data to do that. It shouldn't have been a Schedule 1 drug, because that preordains it to be seen as not having any medical benefit.

We've come a long way from the *Reefer Madness* days, when the public presumed pot was a dangerously addictive psychotic. Why do you think the country has become more and more accepting of cannabis, especially when it comes to medical use?
One reason that's a little less obvious is that there's a bit of distrust in big pharmaceutical companies, along with a desire to find things that are more natural and less toxic that can provide relief. And not just as a substitute but as something that can really work. Within the medical world, there had been resistance to anything that doesn't come out of gleaming, shining labs, which have all sorts of controls on what they do. As we began to experience the opioid epidemic and noticed the data for opioid deaths was down in states allowing medical use [of marijuana], people could accept cannabis as valuable for pain relief.

Based on what you've learned since writing your essay, what are the most effective uses of medical marijuana?
Epilepsy is a big one. We're also seeing a lot of data around its effectiveness with chronic inflammatory

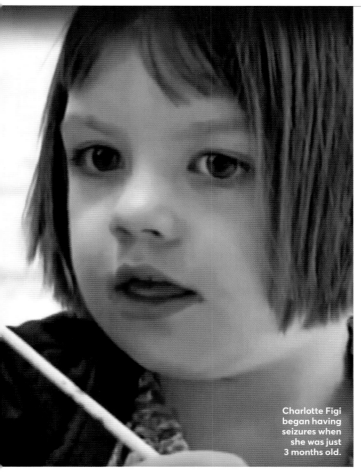

Charlotte Figi began having seizures when she was just 3 months old.

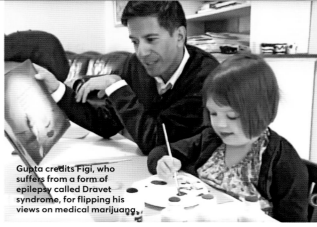

Gupta credits Figi, who suffers from a form of epilepsy called Dravet syndrome, for flipping his views on medical marijuana.

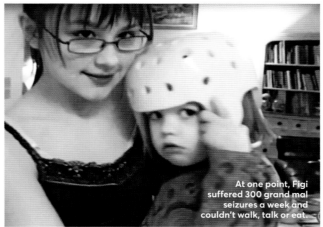

At one point, Figi suffered 300 grand mal seizures a week and couldn't walk, talk or eat.

diseases and autoimmune diseases like rheumatoid arthritis. There seem to be some pretty significant anti-inflammatory effects, mainly in the brain and gut but also in areas such as the joints. We create our own natural cannabinoid receptors in our bodies that can activate the receptors in those areas. When it comes to neuropathic pain and modulating the central nervous system, there's something there. There are also some early-stage studies on medical marijuana's effect on post-traumatic stress disorder that seem promising.

There are so many different ways now for patients to consume medical marijuana—by vaping, in gummies, sodas, oils, creams and soaps—besides just smoking it. Do any of these delivery methods pose a particular danger?
It's still the Wild West out there, in a lot of ways. Smoking it is a concern as opposed to vaping, if you are having lung problems. I've read a bit about vaping and learned that once you start to heat cannabis to a certain temperature, you tend to release other substances that could be problematic or take away

vehicles that allow ingredients to be transported through the body. The use of gummies concerns me, because this isn't a toy we're talking about. There's a confluence between medicinal and recreational use of marijuana, and it's a bit of a spurious argument to say there isn't. I wouldn't say, for instance, that I'm worried about Lipitor being used recreationally. They're not making gummies for Lipitor.

Medical marijuana is still illegal on a federal level, even though most states allow some form of its use. Do you think this will change any time soon?
Right now, we still have this really bizarre federal-state system—and it may worsen, given the views of this administration. This is an issue, because when there is a system where you don't have a consistent way of controlling and verifying what people are using, the market can be flooded with poorly grown or contaminated substances. One of the things I've learned since we started making these CNN documentaries is that medical marijuana deserves to be studied like any other substance—and it will be disappointing if the federal government does not give it that chance.

As the states continue to open up their laws regarding medical cannabis, are there any things consumers should be wary of?
The downside is we don't know exactly what doses to give people. We also don't know whether what they're getting is contaminated or reliable. For example, Charlotte Figi's mom had to do a lot of that research on her own to find what was right for her daughter. That meant going to a particular grow field and finding exactly what CBD level the marijuana had. This is stuff individuals have to do on their own, and that's not how the medicines we respect should be used.

What has been the reaction to your documentaries?
I've had calls from people from all walks of life. There was a judge in New York, who doesn't want to

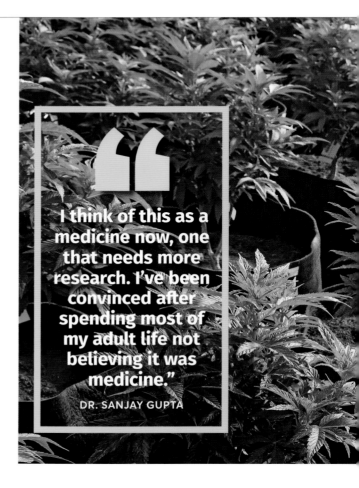

> "I think of this as a medicine now, one that needs more research. I've been convinced after spending most of my adult life not believing it was medicine."
>
> DR. SANJAY GUPTA

be identified, and he was crying on the phone. He was horrified not only about what he had done, putting people away for marijuana use, but because his mother had gone through horrible pain from cancer. She had been totally wigged out on morphine—and he wished he'd seen [medical marijuana] as an option for her. Even in the medical community, I didn't get people who said to me, "You're wrong!" For the most part, people said they'd take a closer look. It was worth doing the homework, spending late nights looking at papers and saying, "Let me dissect this data further and not jump to conclusions."

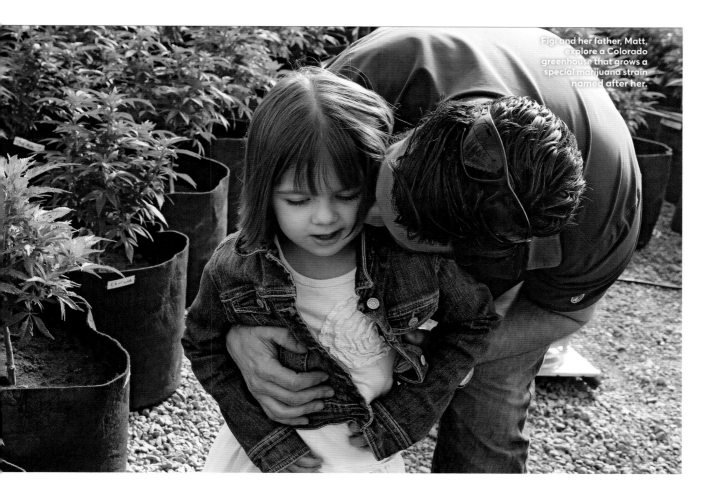

Figi and her father, Matt, explore a Colorado greenhouse that grows a special marijuana strain named after her.

Given all the evidence you've discovered over the past ten years, how would you advise someone who might still be hesitant to see medical marijuana as an option for treatment?

I think of this as a medicine now—but it's one that needs more research, as is always the case with medicine. I have been convinced, after spending most of my adult life not believing marijuana was medicine. Today, not only do I think it has true medicinal value, but I'm convinced it offers value when other medications can't. You just have to be careful—and, even in states where selling it is legal, you still have to do your research to make sure it's safe.

Not to go to the worst-case scenario here, but we are in the middle of an opioid epidemic, and drug overdoses are now considered to be the number-one cause of unintentional death in America. Every demographic in the developed world has increased its life expectancy in recent years, except certain demographics in the United States. I am not suggesting that marijuana is safe and good for people whose brains are still developing, but it is certainly worth taking a hard look at for everyone else.

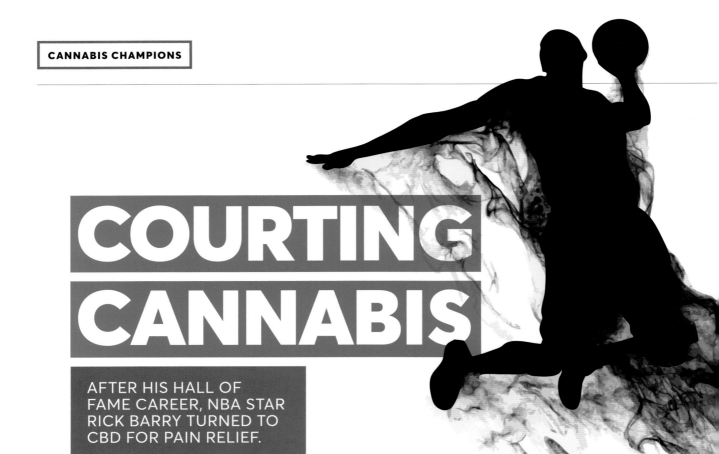

COURTING CANNABIS

AFTER HIS HALL OF FAME CAREER, NBA STAR RICK BARRY TURNED TO CBD FOR PAIN RELIEF.

 Throughout his basketball career, Rick Barry always seemed to be breaking new ground.

He is the only player ever to win a scoring championship in the NCAA, the NBA and the now-departed American Basketball Association. And he was nearly perfect with his free throws, thanks to an idiosyncratic "granny style" underhand toss–and eventually ended up in the NBA's Hall of Fame.

Barry did a lot when he played ball, but one thing he never got around to doing was marijuana. He retired in 1980, and, until a year ago, he'd never used cannabis recreationally or medically. That's when the pain he'd long endured from multiple knee injuries became too much.

He tried THC-free CBD products to help with pain relief, and they worked so well, he's now a major proponent who thinks medical marijuana may help a lot of suffering athletes. Barry now works with Folium Biosciences, the world's largest producer, manufacturer and distributor of THC-free CBD. We spoke with him about how he became a believer.

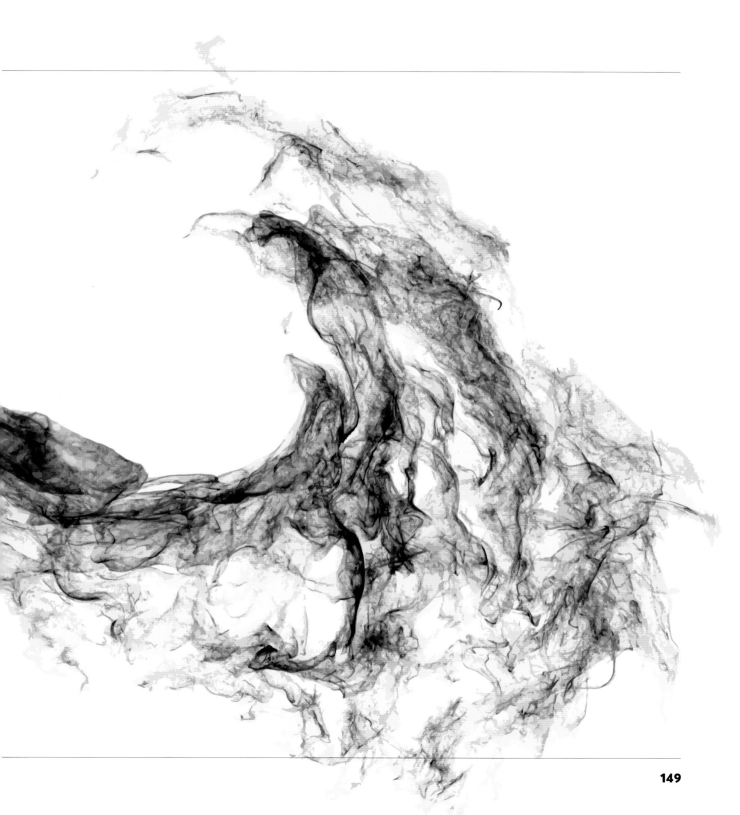

The first time you ever heard of marijuana was after you started your basketball career with the San Francisco Warriors during the 1960s. What were your thoughts on cannabis then, and what are they now?

Obviously, back then, it was when people wanted to get a buzz, and there wasn't much research on medical benefits. It was a totally different world; I did nothing working out then, compared to the sophistication in the training of athletes today. But there's a lot more that can be done in terms of CBD, which is THC-free, and medical marijuana in the NBA. It's still in the Stone Age as far as opiates, not even realizing there are benefits to cannabis. Between medical marijuana and CBD, why in the world wouldn't you do that when you read all the problems with addiction and opiates? It's beyond my comprehension.

So why are opiates prescribed so freely when there is a more-natural, healthier, less-risky alternative?

There's huge money to be made, that's why. Here's the other thing that's crazy. I had a bicycle accident three years ago, and [I was put on] OxyContin. I'd fractured my pelvis in five places, and was in a wheelchair for three months. I told [the doctors] I wanted off this as quickly as possible. Why in the world are you giving me this? I didn't know as much about CBD then, but I would have demanded it if I had. Another thing is that when you get a prescription, they give you way more than you need. You want to have as little as possible.

You did some coaching after you retired. Would you have minded if you found out your players were using medical marijuana?

If someone is hurt, I would be adamant to never put any of my players on opioids. If they needed something, I would want them to try [CBD/medical marijuana] first and see if it works. And if there are other opportunities, based on the research that something would work, obviously use it–truly, totally and completely from a medical point.

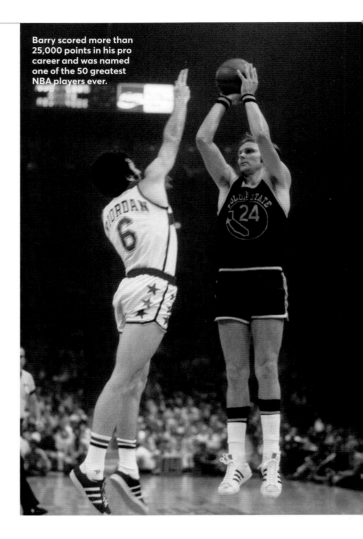

Barry scored more than 25,000 points in his pro career and was named one of the 50 greatest NBA players ever.

Why do you think there is such a stigma to using CBD or medical marijuana?

That shouldn't be an issue. No stigma. You can't overdose, it's not addictive and it's natural. Why in the world is CBD classified as a Schedule 1 drug? It's insane. I can understand it being classified as a drug because of the THC. That's why it's important to understand just how much THC is beneficial from a medical standpoint and what it's beneficial for. If

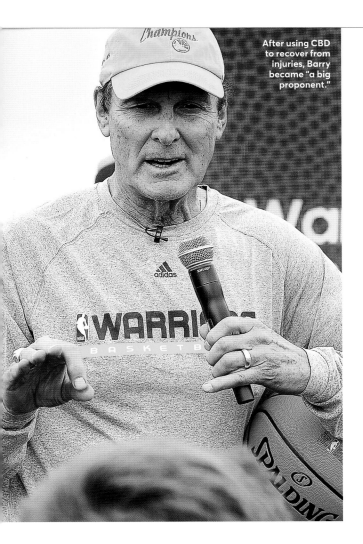

After using CBD to recover from injuries, Barry became "a big proponent."

Do you think that it is becoming more mainstream in sports in general and the NBA in particular?
Let's be realistic. A lot of guys doing it had no idea that marijuana had medical benefits. But I think that as it is even more researched and looked at, it is being used properly and not taken advantage of. I think it is becoming more mainstream...not mainstream, really, because it is at its infancy, but it is being recognized as something that should be given serious consideration.

How did you get involved in this movement?
I was called to help a young man with a brain tumor in Colorado to get playoff tickets with the Warriors. I helped do that, and I heard back from his father. He told me how grateful he was, what it meant to his family, that they had a great time, and he also told me he's involved with this business with CBD. He invited me to visit the plant. When I visit, he tells me what's happening. He says, "I'd love to give you the opportunity to get involved." It's called Folium Biosciences. I told him I wished I'd known about this when I had the bike accident.

CBD's had incredible results, for example, in kids with autism. There are 6 million families with an autistic child, and we're making CBD available at a reasonable cost. When I started looking into this, I wanted to know enough about it to talk about it reasonably intelligently–and it blew me away. I'm hoping to get these things available to people. I want people to open their eyes, get their head out of the proverbial sand and see that there's something to it.

using marijuana can help people, whether it's PTSD or some other condition, then I'm all for it.

Why do you use CBD?
I had two knee surgeries while playing and two after. I hurt my back lifting a rock doing yard work after I had retired. It has never been the same since. I use it for my back when needed. [And of my] knee operations, two were before the new, less-invasive surgery.

What do you hope for in the future?
I'm hoping the research continues. I used to say when I was coaching, "Learn everything you can about this and never stop learning." When you're trying to become a great athlete, you have to learn the basics; without them, you can't improve. You have to build on that foundation. The same is true of this. Stay on top of it. Learn and build on what you know.

BUYING THE FARM

WITH HIS NEW BUSINESS VENTURE, JIM BELUSHI IS EXPANDING FROM HOLLYWOOD INTO WEED.

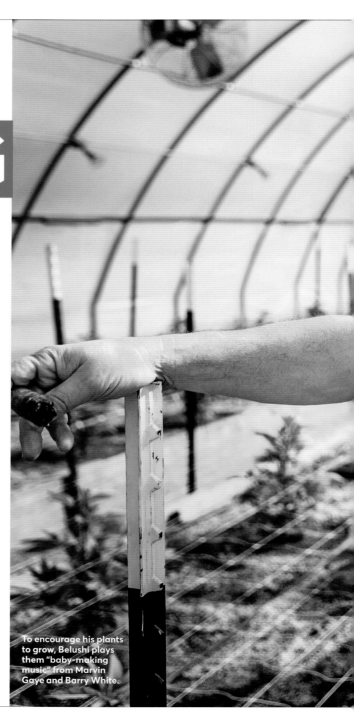

To encourage his plants to grow, Belushi plays them "baby-making music" from Marvin Gaye and Barry White.

Sure, Jim Belushi is a funny guy. After all, whether it was his days on *Saturday Night Live*, his work in movies like *About Last Night...* and *Jingle All the Way* or starring in the long-running sitcom *According to Jim*, comedy has been his thing. However, his new career in cannabis is anything but a laughing matter.

It all began more than four years ago, when Belushi launched a 48-plant medical grow on his 93-acre spread near Eagle Point, Oregon. He dubbed

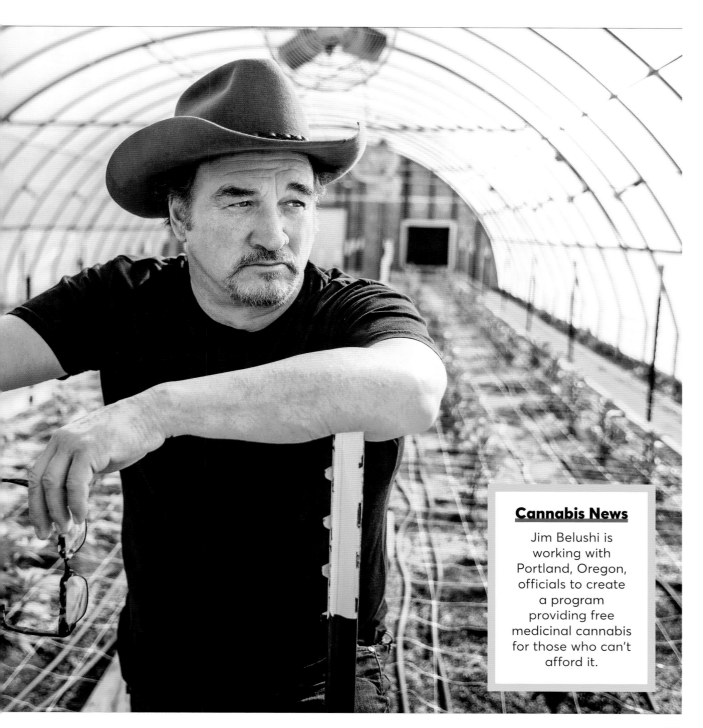

Cannabis News

Jim Belushi is working with Portland, Oregon, officials to create a program providing free medicinal cannabis for those who can't afford it.

it Belushi's Farm, and the land is now home to a 22,000-square-foot licensed grow. His cannabis is just being sold at dispensaries around Oregon, but Belushi has big plans to get his product into the hands of medical and recreational marijuana users across the country. Growing weed may not replace performing as his passion in life, but it's certainly become his new mission.

"There's definitely been a shift in my thinking the past three or four years when it comes to marijuana, thanks to all the discoveries that have been made about the amazing properties of this beautiful plant," says the 65-year-old actor/comedian. "The plants I grow are just like light for the body, and what's wrong with light? Light raises your consciousness and brings your body to good health. This is a spiritual and medical plant that can change our communities."

We spoke with Belushi to learn more about his past, present and future with pot, as well as why he thinks cannabis could have saved his brother John's life.

Was marijuana something you grew up using?

I smoked in high school, between 1968 and 1972. I'm an old hippie who grew up in a white, evangelist suburb of Chicago. We moved to Wheaton from the West Side because my dad didn't want us to be in gangs. It had been voted the All-American City at one point, and I think *I* was the crime rate in Wheaton. So there we were, this ethnic family in the middle of a place like that. My brother John adapted really quickly. He was straight as an arrow in his corduroy pants, V-neck sweater and collared shirt. He was in Honor Society, the football star, the homecoming king. He adapted. I was the troublemaker.

The stigma back then for marijuana was terrible. I didn't pay attention to it, though. My high school was filled with weed. It was a fun thing to do, but as I got into theater and acting, all that kind of fell away because I'd never do anything to get in the way of my performances. I think there were nine years there where I didn't even drink a beer or even think about it. I got busy with life.

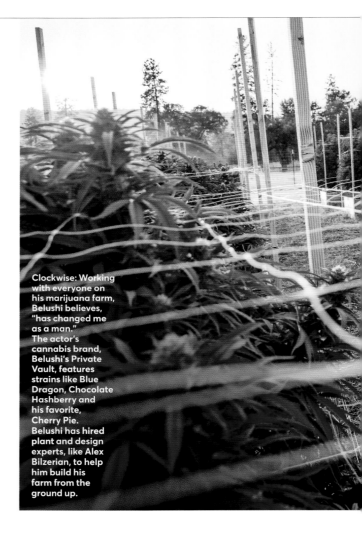

Clockwise: Working with everyone on his marijuana farm, Belushi believes, "has changed me as a man." The actor's cannabis brand, Belushi's Private Vault, features strains like Blue Dragon, Chocolate Hashberry and his favorite, Cherry Pie. Belushi has hired plant and design experts, like Alex Bilzerian, to help him build his farm from the ground up.

John may have been the straight arrow, but he eventually passed away due to a drug overdose. Do you remember seeing a change in him at some point?
I still remember seeing him have a seizure in his senior year of high school. I was in our living room watching TV. He had this little TV on in the kitchen that was really loud. I thought he was being an ass, so I went in there to tell him to turn it down. He wasn't in the kitchen, but I found him in the laundry room

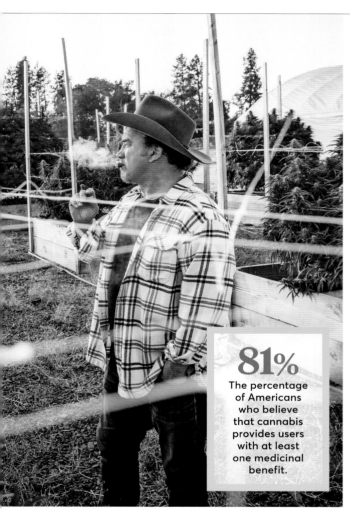

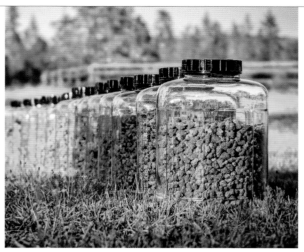

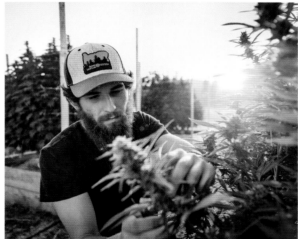

81%

The percentage of Americans who believe that cannabis provides users with at least one medicinal benefit.

holding onto the sink, and he was shaking. I went, "C'mon, John, just turn the TV down," but he was shaking so bad that he fell down. Our mom came in and was able to pull his tongue out of his mouth to keep him from choking. They ended up doing spinal taps on him. They did X-rays. They couldn't find anything. However, I think he was already suffering from the effects of CTE (chronic traumatic encephalopathy) from playing football. He had the most tackles for the team every year, and a lot of the behavior he exhibited was the same as what's been described these many years later for someone suffering with CTE. That's why I really believe that when John had his first joint, it was like medicine for him. And he really needed that medicine. I really believe if we knew then what we know now about cannabis, a lot more people would be alive today. Including my brother.

It's getting more difficult all the time to find someone who doesn't have a story about how his or her life has been touched by the use of medical marijuana. Is that something you've seen as well since jumping into this business?

As I entered into the world of this plant, I discovered more and more amazing moments. For instance, there was the veteran living on the Oregon coast who came up to me teary-eyed to say he was a medic in Iraq, where he saw things happen to the human body nobody should ever see. His PTSD was so bad, he couldn't talk to his children. He couldn't sleep. Then he said my Black Diamond OG was the only medicine he found that would allow him to talk to his kids and get sleep. He hugged me and I said, "I didn't make it man," and he said, "No, but you're the steward."

How important has it been in your life?

I just put CBD ointment on my son's back last night because it was sore. I rub it on my daughter's back when she has cramps. My mother-in-law's knees hurt so I bring her tinctures. She's 79, and has Fox News blasting 24 hours a day. She's the most conservative woman I know, but she uses it. My stepfather-in-law was passing, and they kept giving him morphine, so I gave him a [cannabis] candy bar instead. It didn't heal him, but it created a quality of life where he could talk to us. Wouldn't it be nice to talk to your family as they go rather than having them in this blurred high? It's such a beautiful medicine in that way.

And I always carry my Cherry Pie vape pen with me because of my wife. I would argue with her and then take one little hit off the pen without her noticing. It changed the conversation because it brings you an empathetic heart. It takes away all the things that aren't necessary in life, like having to be right all the time. That's why I call this Cherry Pie the Right Buster. It helps you see what best serves your relationships, whether it's marriage or friendship or work. You don't have to be the one who's right anymore. You see it's just not important.

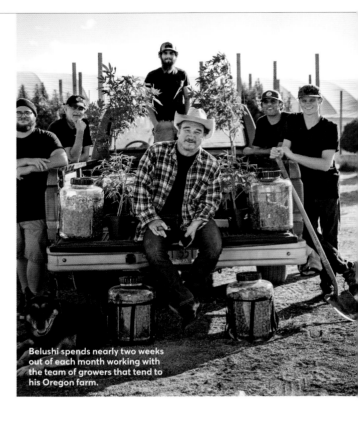

Belushi spends nearly two weeks out of each month working with the team of growers that tend to his Oregon farm.

Several celebrities have started up their own cannabis businesses—Willie Nelson, Tommy Chong and Snoop Dogg, for instance—but they had a reputation with the plant beforehand. What's the key to establishing yourself in this world?

The interest generated within the big business of cannabis is for authenticity, so celebrities that want to just slap their name on a product have been getting turned down. The cannabis business community sees through that quickly, and the consumer sees through it too. I once met a girl who said, "I'd buy something if it had Tupac's name on it." I said, "If you were standing at a counter and saw something with his image on it and you love him, what's your next thought? It's, 'Who's making money off Tupac?'" There's

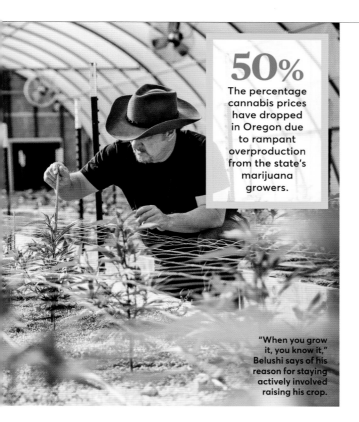

50%

The percentage cannabis prices have dropped in Oregon due to rampant overproduction from the state's marijuana growers.

"When you grow it, you know it," Belushi says of his reason for staying actively involved raising his crop.

Four years ago, I started asking how do I grow this? What do I plant? Everyone in that community helped me. I have a grower there, Captain Jack, who knows everything and has taught me everything. He has been growing since the '60s. I just kept learning. Day 21, learn pruning and keep light going. Day 42, you prune again. It shocks the plant, and draws more THC up. What do you want to know? I'll tell you. I can't believe I'm a farmer!

I recently got offered an acting project, and I asked what the dates for it were. They told me, and I went, "Uh oh, I'm harvesting." They said, "What are you talking about? So we have to block out harvest days in your schedule?" I said, "Yeah I have to be there to pull the plants." I'm clipping it, I'm hanging it, I'm drying it. I have a little tool to measure moisture in buds. I crack the stem to check it. Then I'm involved in the marketing, finding the right graphics for products. I'm learning everything.

What new products are you developing for your Belushi's Private Vault brand?

For now, our flower is available in Oregon dispensaries. We recently introduced joint packs. I'm working on a variety of edibles and am in discussion about maybe doing a beer. I've had talks about doing sublinguals, those little things you drop in your mouth and they melt. Still, always underneath all of this, I'm working for the medicine that CBD provides. I am always trying to find the right product to deliver that.

Given your success in Hollywood, you really don't need to do any of this. So what drives you to stick with the cannabis business?

If you can work with something that can heal people and families, why not jump on it and make it happen? That's what got me here and keeps me here. This plant is something I believe in so deeply. You have to think about money in life, but I always lead with my passion. And what taught me to follow the passion? The cannabis itself, and the enlightenment that comes with it.

no authenticity there. The celebrity piece of this wasn't intentional for me, but I have people from all over saying they're really glad I can bring a voice to the movement. I tell them, "This is a movement? I didn't know. I'm just following the medicine, man!"

How much time do you spend on your farm?

I'm up there about 10 days a month unless it's harvest time, in which case it's a lot longer. I go back and forth a lot. Let's just say this: Everyone in the Medford, Oregon, airport knows me now.

How has starting this business changed your life?

I'm a damn farmer now! I'm fighting rustic mites and aphids. I'm flushing out the irrigation system.

TAKING THE LEAD

BELOVED TELEVISION PERSONALITY MEHMET OZ IS ONE OF THE WORLD'S MOST VISIBLE CHAMPIONS OF MEDICAL MARIJUANA. JUST DON'T ASK HIM TO INHALE.

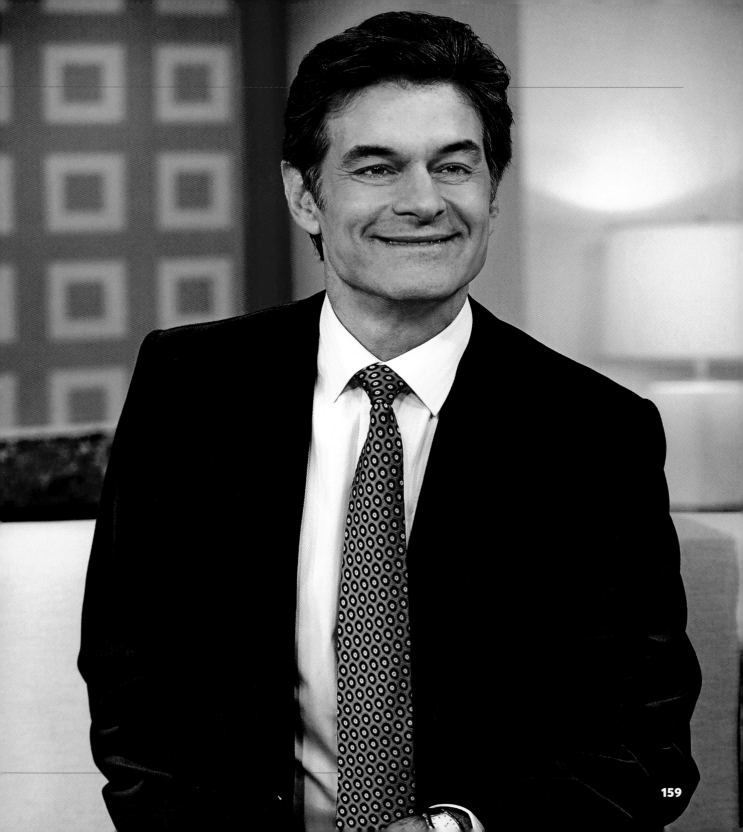

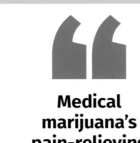

Dr. Mehmet Oz is an absolute buzz-master when it comes to manipulating the cycles of social media and tabloid television. He swears, however, that he's never copped a buzz.

"Just to be clear, I've never smoked a joint in my life," he tells me, in the clipped tones that have mesmerized his many fans. "I've never gotten high. I'm not an advocate of marijuana for recreational reasons, but I think that the evidence supporting the medical benefits of marijuana is clear."

A Harvard-educated cardiothoracic surgeon, Oz's word carries tremendous influence. His popular television and online broadcasts have garnered multiple Emmy awards, reaching more than 2 million viewers with a single episode. In 2008, *Esquire* magazine named him one of the 75 most important people of the 21st century.

So in championing medical marijuana over the past few years, Oz has played a key role in the growing acceptance of cannabis across America's vast heartland. He's even been able to spread the good word for weed in the Trump White House.

■ CANNABIS CONVERT

The doctor's well-publicized belief in the plant's healing properties was inspired in part by the stories of his friends, such as billionaire sports entrepreneur Ed Snider.

"He developed a very bad bladder cancer and was dying," Oz tells me. "He was in terrible pain. The doctors were giving him opiates and opioids that wouldn't work—all the usual things you usually do for cancer patients. And this nurse said, 'I know you're a straight-up guy, but if you'd be willing to try just a little bit of marijuana, it might help take the edge off the pain. And maybe you won't be completely out of it on opiates.' So, he tried medical marijuana. It had a dramatic impact, and he lived a year without pain. His daughter, Lindy, has become one of medical marijuana's biggest advocates, and this is a blue-blood family from Philadelphia."

Pain and suffering are no respecters of the class system, and the TV doc found that elites were just as much in need of the healing powers of cannabis as some of the less well-heeled guests on his program.

"I hear stories like this over and over again," he says. "Like my close friend Montel Williams. Here's a man who served his nation in the Navy, and then was told by that nation that his intractable multiple

> **Medical marijuana's pain-relieving power can help break the opioid crisis."**
>
> DR. MEHMET OZ

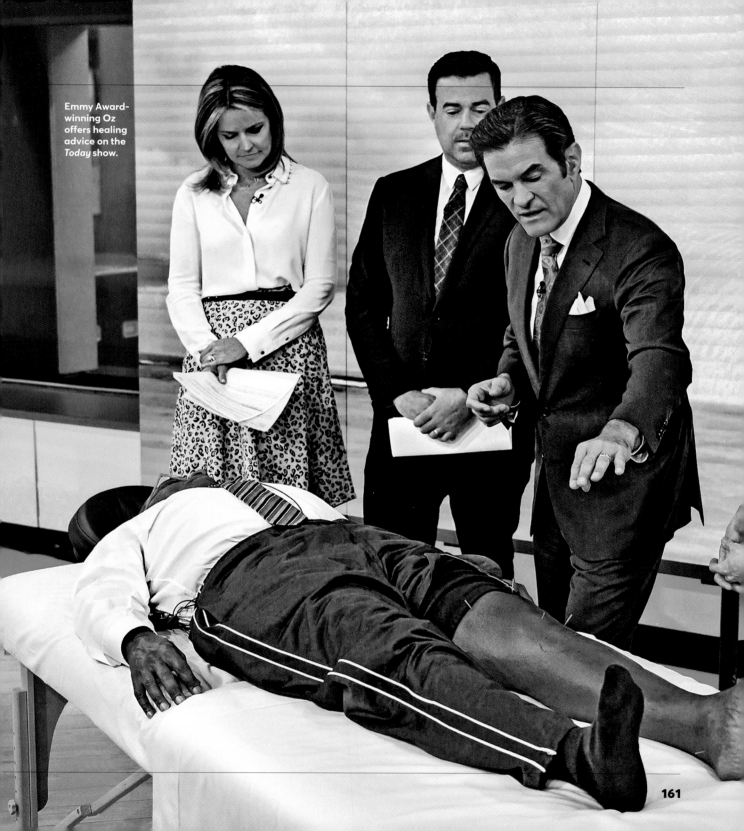

Emmy Award-winning Oz offers healing advice on the *Today* show.

161

sclerosis pain could not be alleviated. Now he can't get out of bed without marijuana. He's become an advocate and has taught me a lot about it. He took me to dispensaries, and also where they grow the pot. Also, I've had guests on my show with children who have had seizures and experienced a complete remission of symptoms, thanks to medical marijuana."

The doctor has been particularly vocal about the efficacy of cannabis as an alternative to opioid drugs such as fentanyl for pain relief. "Medical marijuana's pain-relieving power can help break the opioid crisis," he states. "I realized there's been a massive fraud in pain treatment. There was so much money being made using opioids to treat pain that there was almost a purposeful silence about other options. Nobody would research meditation, physical activity and things like medical marijuana for pain management."

■ Cannabis Needs to Be Medicine

The Dr. Oz Show has done much to fuel the CBD mania. But his personal response to the phenomenon is more muted. "I'm encouraged by it," he says, "but it's basically a work-around. CBD can be harvested from hemp, which is grown legally. But CBD is often more effective when there's a little bit of THC in the product. And that can only come from the marijuana plant. The terpenes in marijuana are also important. This needs to be medicine. It should be declassified and regulated by the FDA with very clear definitions of what percentage of CBD, THC and terpenes are recommended for specific medical conditions. If you have a headache, use this. If you have insomnia, use that. I can't recommend marijuana without knowing which strains are effective. I can't just prescribe Blue Kush any more than I could prescribe a 2014 merlot for a certain medical condition."

In 2018, Donald Trump appointed Oz to the President's Council on Sports, Fitness & Nutrition. This allowed the physician to speak with different agencies about declassifying cannabis as a Schedule 1 drug. "Nobody wants it to be Schedule 1," he said in a 2018 interview. "The FDA thinks it should be regulated.

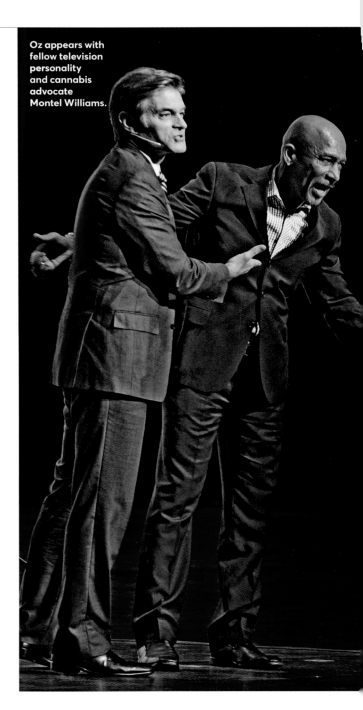

Oz appears with fellow television personality and cannabis advocate Montel Williams.

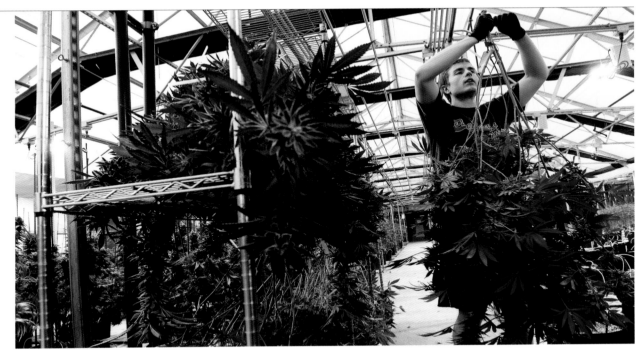

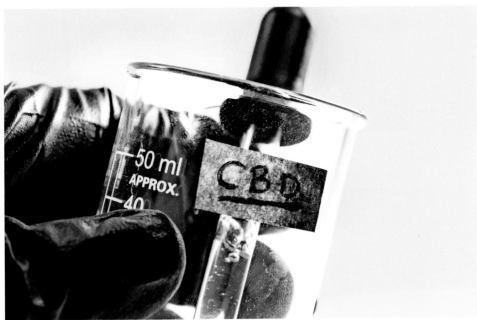

Above: A Canadian grow technician manicures a plant that is helping to put his country at the forefront of what could be a $150 billion-plus global market.
Left: CBD oil extract made from cannabis flower.

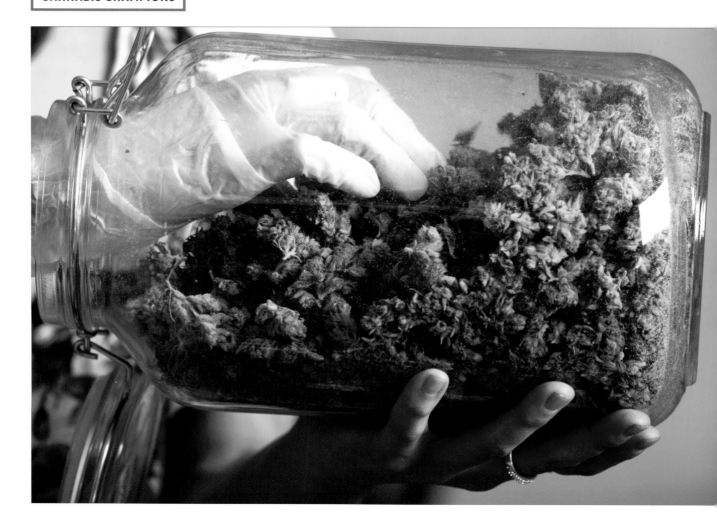

They don't think it should be Schedule 1. The DEA figures the DOJ [Department of Justice] doesn't want it around. Everyone is trying to figure everyone else out. Nobody wants to be on the hook for it. We need strong leadership that calls a spade a spade."

■ Learning From His Viewers

Oz has already received a clearer directive from his millions of viewers and social media followers. Their support for cannabis legalization has been, he says, "overwhelmingly positive. There's a danger to society when people realize there's a law that's hypocritical. They stop following the law in general. An unfair law is very dangerous for a country. There may be a law that I don't like, but if I understand the rationale for it I can respect it. But if a country passes a law that has so little merit, it undermines all the laws that are fair. Where do you draw the line?"

Oz feels confident that Big Pharma–rather than Big Tobacco, major food and beverage companies

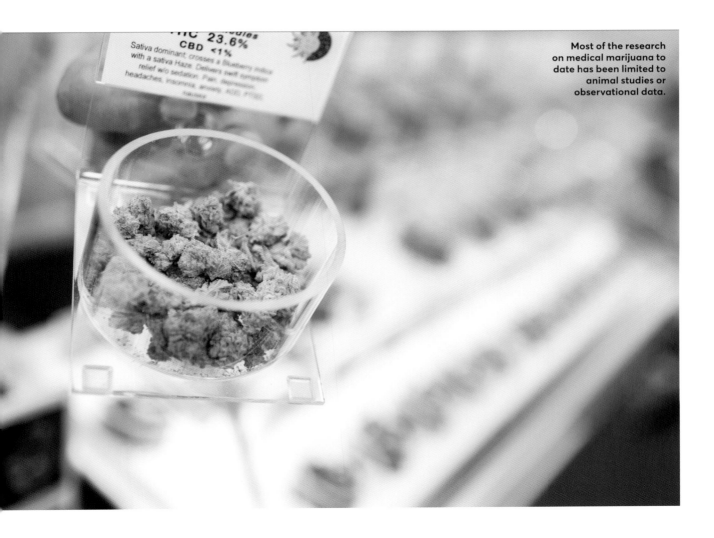

THC 23.6%
CBD <1%

Sativa dominant, crosses a Blueberry indica with a sativa Haze. Delivers swift complete relief w/o sedation. Pain, depression, headaches, insomnia, anxiety, ADD, PTSD.

Most of the research on medical marijuana to date has been limited to animal studies or observational data.

and others who are now flocking to the cannabis space in large numbers–will eventually be the industry that will come to control the lucrative marijuana marketplace.

"Pharma is already making inroads," he says, "and the smaller companies that are good are going to get bought. But unfortunately, American companies are way behind. Canadian companies are already producing products that will satisfy the huge U.S. demand, once our legal system catches up

with the rest of the world. Most countries around the world won't allow marijuana, but the countries that are allowing the research–like Israel and Canada–they're going to be ahead. I think we need to move [cannabis] out of Schedule 1 and allow our researchers free reign."

Looking ahead, Oz predicts that cannabis change will be swift. "And when the resistance crumbles," he says, "it's going to go down like the Berlin Wall. It's ripe for a crash."

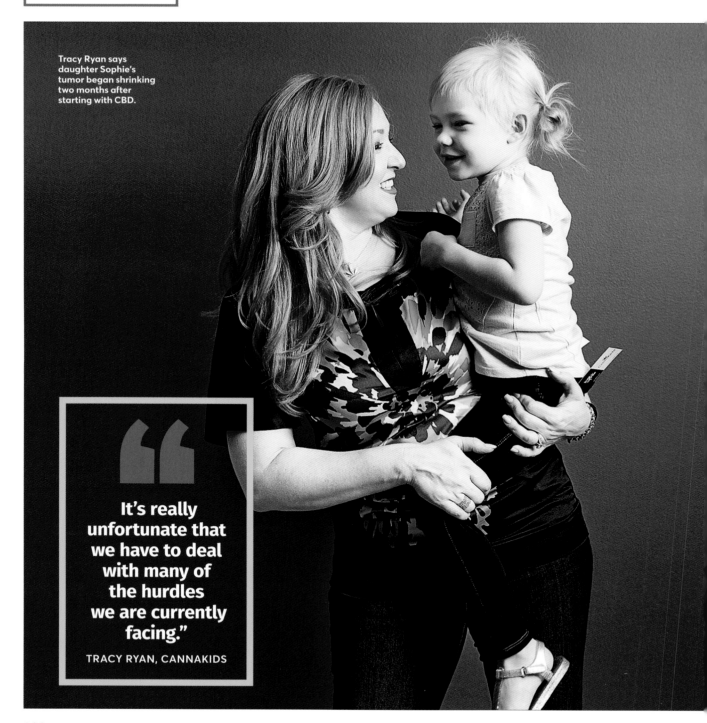

Tracy Ryan says daughter Sophie's tumor began shrinking two months after starting with CBD.

"It's really unfortunate that we have to deal with many of the hurdles we are currently facing."

TRACY RYAN, CANNAKIDS

A MOTHER'S FIGHT

HOW FOUR MOMS ARE SAVING THEIR CHILDREN WITH THE HELP OF CANNABIS.

Tracy Ryan's life changed in the blink of an eye. Literally.

In 2013, she'd noticed a shaking in her 8-month-old daughter Sophie's left eyeball. A chain of doctors' appointments later, Tracy was informed that her baby girl had an optic pathway glioma, a slow-growing tumor that can cause cancer and, in some cases, death. Chemotherapy was the only option for treatment.

The type of tumor Sophie suffered from had a survival rate of 90 percent but also a recurrence rate of 85 percent. As the Ryans searched for any alternatives for Sophie, they connected with TV host Ricki Lake, who was making a documentary called *Weed the People* about the use of cannabis oil for pediatric diseases. That led to Sophie starting on cannabis oils as well as chemotherapy, which drastically improved her condition.

The experience not only saved the girl's life, it also inspired Tracy to start CannaKids, a California cooperative corporation that provides information as well as medicinal cannabis oils to ill children and adults. She spoke with us about her journey and how she's translated the trauma into a triumph.

"The wrenching desperation led me, my husband and Sophie on a roller-coaster ride of despair and discovery, of cancer and chemotherapy and, most surprising, of cannabis. At first, Sophie's neurosurgeon told us that we needed to prepare for full blindness. There was a 100 percent chance of her losing sight in her left eye, and, best-case scenario, she would have minimal vision in her right eye," Tracy says.

■ "IT NEEDS TO STOP NOW"

"When I first started this process, I was lucky enough to meet Ricki Lake and [her producing partner] Abby Epstein, who were making a documentary about using cannabis oil to treat pediatric illnesses. They were able to really guide me through and bring me oils. I think it was around $7,000 of free oils they had, originally, procured for another little girl, who'd left to go to a legal state. I was lucky enough to get those.

"There are children in this optic pathway glioma group that I'm a member of on Facebook who have literally been in chemotherapy for 13 years. So, again, this is why I'm so passionate about working with universities and other very respected pediatric hospitals around the country. I can get answers for my child, and I can get research going in Israel on her brain-tumor sample. I can get answers for my kid so that she doesn't have to be one of those kids who goes through 13 years of chemotherapy. That sort of thing needs to stop, and it needs to stop now.

"Honestly, other patients are dying. If a child gets cancer in Jamaica, that child is sent home with a morphine drip if the parents can't afford the out-of-pocket expense of chemotherapy. It's sad to see some of these regions and what these patients are going through—but it's also enlightening to see that their governments are getting behind them...and getting behind cannabis.

"It's really unfortunate that we have to deal with many of the hurdles we have to deal with currently and the federal regulations that are putting up roadblocks. Our government is going to have to get onboard. We're supposed to be the greatest country in the world, yet we are exponentially behind on this initiative.

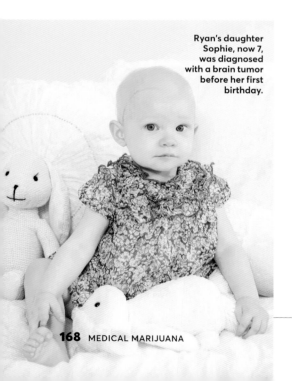

Ryan's daughter Sophie, now 7, was diagnosed with a brain tumor before her first birthday.

"Recently, though, I have to say the conversation really is changing. There was an article published on forbes.com titled "Medical Marijuana for Children With Cancer Is Broadly Supported by Doctors." This just goes to show how far we've come in six years' time, since we started this with Sophie. Back then, cannabis was a medicine that doctors had never heard of for children. They had heard of it for glaucoma, for pain or as a drug to get high. But now the masses are really supporting cannabis for pediatri use—and especially for pediatric research.

"Recent results we're seeing for autism are absolutely incredible. I can safely say this is, hands-down, the area in which we've had the most success. It's a really wonderful, beautiful thing when you have a child who was very violent and self-injurious, and they're smiling, happy, giving hugs and letting people touch them, and they haven't had a violent rage—we saw a child that hadn't had a violent rage in two years, who before was not even able to go to school. You can help with a lot of the side effects of autism, which can really create havoc in a family and everyday life as a whole.

■ CREATING CANNAKIDS

"That's why we're so excited about human trials starting now on autism with nonpsychoactive

THCA—the 'a' stands for acid. It's like juicing the raw plant, essentially. The therapeutic value that we're seeing in THCA and CBDA, which has a lot of new reporting behind it, is amazing. We're really trying to get that message out there as well.

"When I started down this path, I had so many people say to me, 'Do not call your company CannaKids. Do not start screaming about pediatric cancer and giving kids pot. They're going to come and take your kid and throw you in jail.' But I just instinctively had this feeling: I can't sit by and keep what I've experienced a secret. I can't sit by and let families suffer. I cannot be afraid of what's going to happen to me, because I believe I'm here for a purpose. My daughter is here for a purpose. And I'm not going to let fear stand in the way of trying to help others. And I'm so happy that I've been able to do this, because it's what initially led me to say yes to everything that we've done since Sophie got sick.

■ A STRONGER, SMILING SOPHIE

"As for her current health, Sophie has another MRI scheduled. She goes to chemo every two weeks, with no side effects from the chemotherapy. The cannabis is not affecting her blood count for the protocol that she's on. She's also in school now; we can't take her out, so she's not traveling as much.

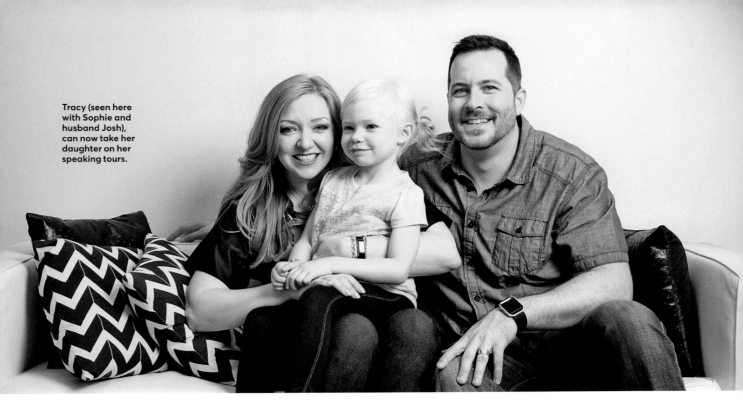

Tracy (seen here with Sophie and husband Josh), can now take her daughter on her speaking tours.

"Whenever she can, though, Sophie comes with me when I travel to speak. She has her own suitcase with wheels that she pulls though the airport. She has her own business cards. When the plane takes off, she says that it tickles her belly. She loves the snacks. She loves watching the movies. She loves napping on the airplane. She's literally the best little travel companion you could ever imagine. Sophie goes all over with me. She and I were at the TMC Innovation Institute, at Texas Medical Center, in Houston. We were speaking at an event, and I brought her up onstage with me at the very end, as I do whenever she travels with me.

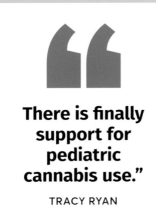

There is finally support for pediatric cannabis use."

TRACY RYAN

"Sophie stepped up to the stage and looked up at me with these big, blue eyes and said, 'Mommy, can I say something?' And I said, 'Of course, you can, honey.' So, she grabbed the microphone from my hand, unprompted, unrehearsed, and said, 'Hi, my name is Sophie, and I take cannabis...' She just brought down the house!

"Sophie was so healthy and vivacious, so energetic–running all around the TMC Medical Incubator, introducing herself to people, telling them to come watch her speak. You can't look at this kid and know that she's been on cannabis since 2013 and believe that anything bad has happened to her. Because it hasn't!"

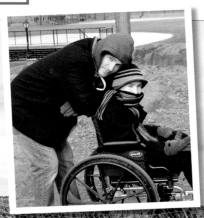

Coltyn, now 20, was in a wheelchair when he and father Tommy (inset) first went to Colorado.

"I THANK GOD EVERY DAY WE FOUND THIS PATH."

It was a decision no parent should ever have to make. And yet, there it was, staring Wendy Turner in the face. Her son Coltyn had been diagnosed with Crohn's disease at age 11, after nearly drowning at a Boy Scout camp and developing a bacterial infection. And, despite trying drugs like Entocort and Humera, his situation was only getting worse: His lymph nodes were swelling to the point where doctors thought he might develop T-cell lymphoma. So, by the time her son was 13, Wendy basically had three options to choose from: She could have Coltyn try another medication that might increase the chance of lymphoma. Or she could allow him to go through surgery that required removing 22 inches of diseased bowel and would leave him with a colostomy bag for the rest of his life. Then, there was a third choice: try some sort of alternative treatment outside the realm of traditional medicine.

■ LOOKING FOR A LIFESAVER

"He was only 13, and there was no way I was putting him through that surgery," recalls Wendy. "Our doctor said we could try alternative treatments, but he couldn't give us any information on them. That was my green light to do more research on cannabis."

As she dug into the subject, Wendy learned of an Israeli study of 21 Crohn's patients who tried medical marijuana. Eleven gained some kind of symptom relief, and nine had complete remission. There didn't seem to be any indication of detrimental side effects, so Wendy's decision was not a difficult one.

"Maybe Coltyn might lose some brain cells, but the treatment wasn't going to faze him," she says. "If he could be hungry and gain weight, have more energy and possibly go into remission...why wouldn't we try this?"

Possibly because first, the Turners lived in Illinois, which

Our doctor said we could try alternative treatments, but he couldn't give us any information on them. That was my green light.

WENDY TURNER

didn't have a comprehensive medical-marijuana law; and second, Wendy was a typical mom who believed "pot was bad for you. We'd even kicked family members out of our lives for smoking it." But given that her son's life was at stake, she let go of the latter concern. As for the former, she solved it by sending her husband with Coltyn to Colorado, where medical marijuana became legal in 2000.

■ "SOMETHING WAS HAPPENING"

They found a caregiver there who started the boy off with some pot brownies and a CBD oil. And within a few days of starting with the brownies, Wendy got a call from her husband.

"He said they got cabin fever in the hotel they had to stay at since we didn't have a house there," she recalls. "They decided to take a trip up into the mountains, and when they got there, Coltyn started throwing snowballs and walking around to see the sights. A couple of weeks before that, he was in a wheelchair. Now he was running in the snow. So right then, we knew something was happening."

When Coltyn and his father returned home to Illinois, Wendy was stunned not only to see color back in his face but also to see him standing in the driveway. Within seven months of that first Colorado trip, he had gone into complete clinical remission–and the Turners were a changed family.

"It spun us around so much that we started speaking out," explains Wendy, noting that the family moved permanently to Colorado to ensure Coltyn's access to cannabis. "We thought it was important to let other kids with Crohn's know they could use this without the side effects that come with other drugs."

To get the word out about his miraculous turnaround, Coltyn started a Facebook page–Coltyn's Crue–that lobbies for more-accessible medical cannabis nationwide and features the now-20-year-old's inspirational thoughts. ("I'd rather be illegally alive than legally dead," reads one of his recent posts.) Wendy will never forget watching him watch Attorney General Jeff Sessions' confirmation hearing in early 2017.

"Coltyn lost it," she says. "Sessions said, 'My job is to uphold the law—and if you don't like the law, change it.' Coltyn heard that and said, 'We're going to Washington to change the law!' And we did go to lobby for change. We're tired of waiting." Still, Wendy is optimistic about the future, because she's already seen it in Coltyn's smiling face.

"Every day, I think about where we'd be if we hadn't found medical cannabis," she explains. "We wouldn't have Coltyn here with us. He'd be dead. If we'd continued on the path we were on, we would have killed him—so I thank God every day we found this other path. Now we have this beautiful young man who is going to change the world."

THE FACTS ABOUT CROHN'S DISEASE

WHAT IS IT?
According to the National Institute of Diabetes and Digestive and Kidney Diseases, Crohn's is a chronic illness that inflames and irritates the digestive tract. It generally starts on a gradual basis but can worsen over time.

WHO GETS IT?
Estimates are that between 500,000 and 700,000 people in the U.S. have Crohn's disease. While it can strike at any age, it is more likely to occur in those who are between 20 and 29, those who have a family member with inflammatory bowel disease, and those who smoke. Research has found that people who have Crohn's disease in their large intestine may be more likely to develop colon cancer.

WHAT ARE THE SYMPTOMS?
Possible indications of Crohn's disease include diarrhea, stomach pain, bleeding from the rectum, fatigue, nausea, constipation and anal bleeding.

WHAT ARE THE COMPLICATIONS?
Those with Crohn's disease may experience intestinal blockage, abscesses, ulcers, anal fissures, malnutrition and inflammation in other areas of the body, such as the joints, eyes and skin.

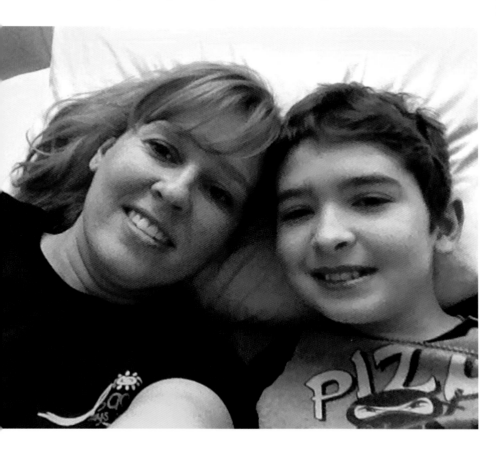

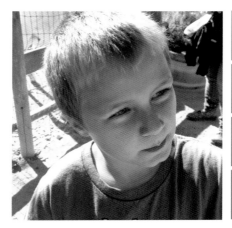

"I'LL DO WHATEVER IS GOING TO HELP MY KIDS."

It's hard enough for a parent to deal with a tragic medical diagnosis for one of their children. So it's almost impossible to imagine what Jennifer Akridge went through after hearing in 2010 that her son, Wyatt, had autism and, three years later, learning that daughter Kayce had cancer. Even worse, by March 2015, 11-year-old Kayce was struggling with not only chemo but also the medications prescribed to combat its side effects, including severe headaches, pain and nausea.

Desperate for help, Akridge decided to contact CannaKids, a group she'd learned about from another parent. That's when she heard founder Tracy Ryan (p. 166) speak about the work being done not only for cancer patients but also for kids with extreme epilepsy and autism. Akridge and her husband met with pediatrician Bonni Goldstein, MD, who specializes in cannabis-oil therapy. After getting the blessing of Kayce's reluctant great-grandmother, the family started Kayce on cannabis treatments after she received the painful chemotherapy for her spine.

"My grandmother got to witness, 10 minutes after Kayce's first dose of cannabis oil, how she was able to keep something down," explains Akridge. "She was able to get up, play and laugh. After 10 minutes! That's after being bedridden. We were like, 'This is it.'"

Wyatt also started on cannabis oils and began to see significant benefits as well. "He was put on three different medications—Risperdal, Vyvance and Zoloft—at 7 years old! The Risperdal helped him sleep, but it also created aggression," says Akridge. "That's the reason I looked for [another] medication. He had gotten to the point where he attacked an 18-month-old, and it was devastating to me."

A MARIJUANA MIRACLE

Kayce has completed chemotherapy and cannabis-oil treatment (for now), and her relieved mom says she is "thriving." Wyatt, meanwhile, stopped conventional psychological medications and is treated exclusively with cannabis oils. He has recovered enough that he can now start attending school.

Jennifer knows that despite the incredible success stories she's heard since working with CannaKids, there are still doubters who are swayed by the stigma. But as far as she is concerned, there's no arguing with the results she's observed firsthand.

"I don't care...I'll do whatever is going to help my kids," she says.

"HE WAS FIGHTING FOR HIS LIFE."

For Amy Dawn Bourlon-Hilterbran, the tiny town of Choctaw, Oklahoma, was more than simply her home; it was a reflection of her identity. A woman of Native American ancestry, her family had lived there for generations. "That was our place, that was our people," she explains. And then, a few years ago, she had to cut ties and leave, because she didn't want her child to die there. In 2014, Bourlon-Hilterbran's son Austin, then 12, was on life support. His organs were failing, the result of the ever-changing pharmaceutical cocktails he'd been prescribed in order to control seizures he'd endured since he was 1 year old. "If the seizures didn't kill him first, the organ damage would likely kill him within two years," Bourlon-Hilterbran says.

Austin had been diagnosed with Dravet syndrome, a severe form of epilepsy for which there is no cure, and the drugs seemed to be causing more damage than relief. He seized daily, and his body was shutting down. With conventional medication no longer an option, Bourlon-Hilterbran went searching for a miracle. There were none to be found in Oklahoma, where medical marijuana was illegal. She and Austin were left with no choice but to look elsewhere, specifically to cannabis-friendly Colorado, which legalized medical use in 2000 and recreational use in 2012. Her husband, Jason, Austin's stepfather (his biological dad died when he was 1), was skeptical of the benefits of cannabis and initially remained in Oklahoma with their two young sons, Nathaniel and Freeman. Alone in an unfamiliar state, Bourlon-Hilterbran didn't know where to turn. "We had no idea if it was going to work," she says. "We didn't get any help, in any direction."

Forced to quickly educate herself, she chose a regimen of THC and THCA (the precursor chemical to THC) for Austin after learning they were the most effective treatments for kids with seizures who'd been on pharmaceuticals long-term. It took 10 months to fully wean Austin from the meds, but the first time he took THCA drops, he went three days without seizing. His mobility and speech began to improve.

"My son has never been as high on cannabis as he was on pharmaceuticals," Bourlon-Hilterbran explains. "He was a zombie who was seizing all the time. Now he's a different young man."

■ A LIFESAVING ROUTINE

The cannabis was working, but living apart from her family took an emotional toll on Bourlon-Hilterbran. After six months, the separation proved to be too much for Jason as well, so he left his job, packed up Nathaniel and Freeman, and joined his wife and an ever-improving Austin in Colorado.

"[Neither of us would] have believed it if we hadn't seen it ourselves," she says. "It has been amazing. Our son goes weeks or months without a seizure. He had autistic tendencies, but not anymore. He's happy again. He can feel one coming on; he can communicate, he knows what he needs to fix it."

These days, Austin's routine includes THC and THCA administered multiple ways—orally, via drops; on his feet, with topical creams; and through suppositories. Bourlon-Hilterbran mixes

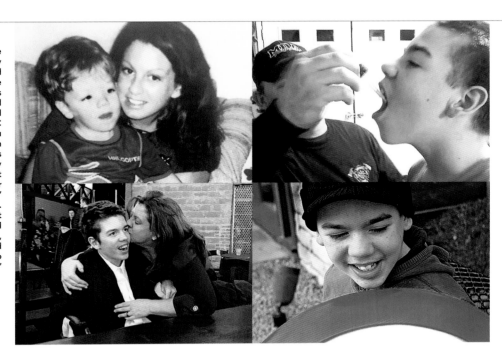

Austin (seen here with mother Amy Dawn) suffered seizures since he was 1 year old. His current medical cannabis ritual includes THC delivered orally via drops. Although her son still has some seizures, Amy Dawn says that his life is "happier and healthier" with cannabis. After Austin spent years on traditional pharmaceuticals, his mother worried they were "going to kill our kid."

up the methods of ingestion to keep her son from building up a tolerance. "We start off with his edible in the morning. He's getting 10 milligrams of THC in the morning. He gets 100 milligrams of a four-compound specialized topical twice a day. He gets Cannatol once a day. He gets CBM once a day. Once a week, we have patches of THCA. If we hit something horrible, we'll get out the full-extract cannabis oil, much like for a cancer patient: 50 grams in 90 days." Austin's seizures haven't entirely disappeared. However, when they strike now, Cannatol intranasal spray, roll-ons and suppositories are administered. The latter

have apparently proven to be the most effective. They are made by Incredibles, a Colorado medical-cannabis company cofounded by Bob Eschino. The way he sees it, he's not just producing medicines. He's bringing families together. "Nothing can convince me cannabis isn't one of the most healing plants on the planet," Eschino says.

■ HELPING FAMILIES FIND HOPE

Now Bourlon-Hilterbran is helping those who are just beginning their journey. She cofounded the American Refugee Foundation (AMRF), which assists families who've moved to Colorado with little more than hope and a prayer.

"People are coming here with terminally ill patients, and it's been too hard to find basic information. I vowed that we were going to change that," she says. AMRF now assists 300 families from 39 states and 30 countries. "We're saving lives every single day," Bourlon-Hilterbran adds.

Ultimately, she knows all too well the high price families pay to uproot in order to treat ill children and has become a fervent advocate for nationwide medical access. "We want everybody to go home," she says. "We want everybody to have access to this plant, regardless of where they live."

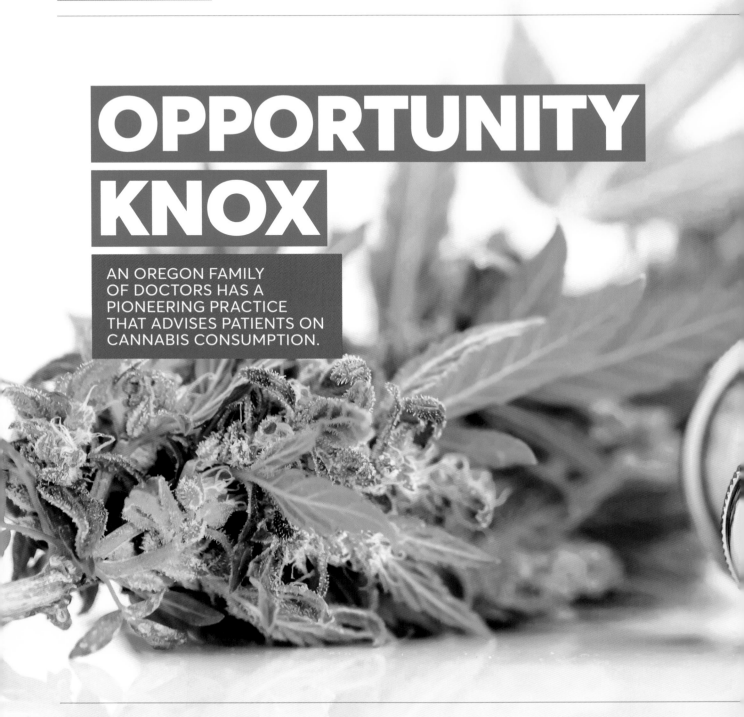

OPPORTUNITY KNOX

AN OREGON FAMILY OF DOCTORS HAS A PIONEERING PRACTICE THAT ADVISES PATIENTS ON CANNABIS CONSUMPTION.

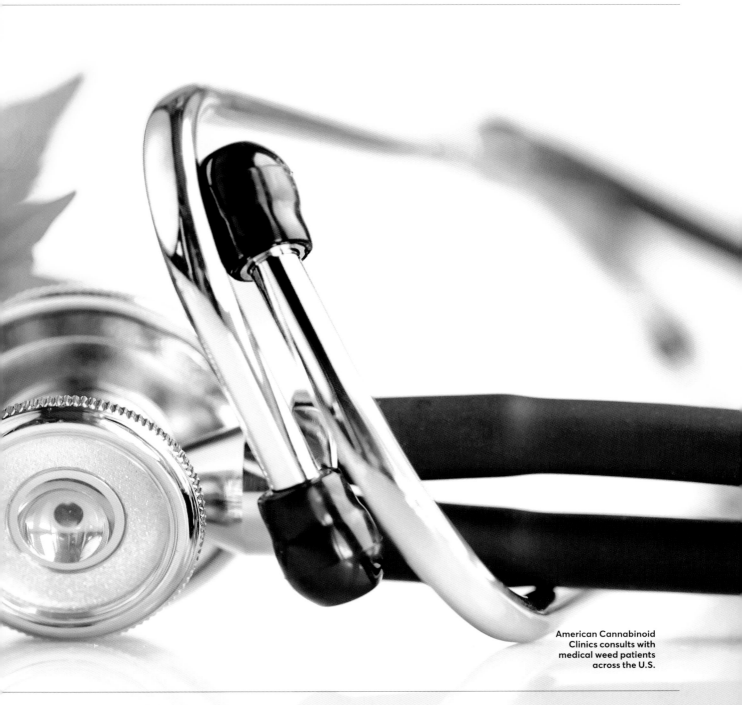

American Cannabinoid
Clinics consults with
medical weed patients
across the U.S.

Most families eventually come up with some way for everyone in the clan to bond. For some, it's an ocean cruise. For others, it's an annual picnic. For still others, it's a simple trip to the cineplex or mall. For the Knoxes, however, it's all about the cannabis.

Husband-and-wife team Drs. David and Janice Knox have launched the Oregon-based American Cannabinoid Clinics, along with their daughters, Drs. Rachel and Jessica Knox. Their practice has offered what they call "integrative endocannabinoid medicine" since 2015, which means they consult with patients about how endocannabinoid medicine can help whatever ails them. The science of CBD is still relatively new, making it difficult to find doctors schooled in the ways of cannabinoids. So the ACC is definitely ahead of the curve when it comes to combining traditional medicine with cannabis-related healing.

"This is a family effort to answer the obvious needs of patients who see cannabis as an alternative to conventional medicine," explains Dr. Janice. "My family and I started out in the traditional medical-card-writing clinics, where it was obvious the patients needed more than the 10 minutes doctors were allowed to spend with them. These patients were looking for health-care providers who help with the safe use of medical marijuana for their many medical problems without being judged. We felt that we could answer this need."

We spoke with her to learn more about the services American Cannabinoid Clinics can provide, and how working in the cannabis field isn't just helping other families—it's also bringing hers closer together.

Has CBD been something your family has incorporated into your practice?

Yes. We practice cannabinoid medicine. We try to use the most appropriate cannabinoid for the medical condition to be addressed. CBD is the new "buzzword" cannabinoid. So this is a great cannabinoid to start most patients off with.

Among the four of you, do you each have a different expertise you bring to cannabinoid medicine?

Dr. David, an emergency room physician, is very scientific in his thinking and brings that perspective. Dr. Rachel, who is in family practice medicine, is not only knowledgeable in the science, but is also the chair of the Oregon Cannabis Commission. She is very involved in policy and regulations concerning medical cannabis in Oregon, and we all hope to influence regulation across the nation. Dr. Jessica is in preventative medicine and very knowledgeable in the science and does a great job on the speaking circuit, helping to establish endocannabinology as a discipline. I am in anesthesiology and love doing the research and thinking about possible formulations that will lead to safer and more efficacious medical therapies.

When you talk to your patients, what is the most common misconception that they have about CBD and cannabis?

Most come in ready to use the products. However, they're looking for ways to take control of their health, and the propaganda about the harms of cannabis still lingers. They're concerned with getting high, needing to smoke and becoming addicted.

What separates ACC from others in the medical-marijuana field?

I don't feel there are others out there doing what we're doing. Our goal is to help others understand that it's the physiology and lifestyle medicine that we are trying to address. It's not just about cannabis. It's about treating medical problems at the root cause and not just the symptoms. If we think and teach holistically, we're treating more than the symptoms of disease.

What are your top three tips for someone seeking to improve their health with CBD?

First, CBD is a great tool—but it needs help. Look to your food and nutrition for your first medicine. Second, look for safe, lab-tested and well-labeled products. Not all CBD product offerings are safe. And don't be afraid of using a ration that has some THC. Third, don't be afraid to adjust the dosage. Start low and go slow to titrate to symptomatic relief. The safety margin is wide.

You are based in Oregon, but if somebody lives in a different (and legal) state, can they still use your services?

We see patients nationally and globally by using our HIPAA-compliant telemedicine platform. They can either call our office or self-schedule at our website [theacclinics.com].

What effect has starting up American Cannabinoid Clinics had on the Knox family?

It's been fantastic. We've always been a close family. The joy of working together in this amazing space is beyond my dreams. The reactions we get from our colleagues, patients and the entire industry are very supportive and encouraging. I think we're a bit of an oddity to everyone, but it's fun.

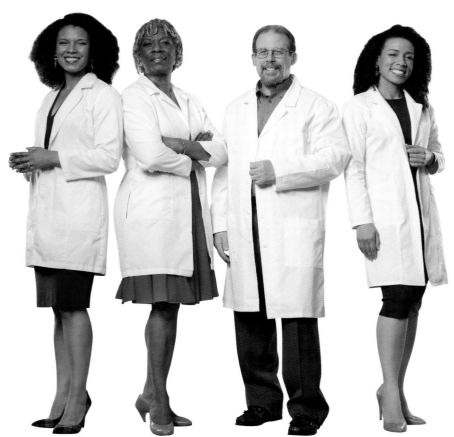

Our goal is to help others understand that it's the physiology and lifestyle medicine that we are trying to address."

DR. JANICE KNOX

ACC is run by the Knoxes: Jessica, Janice, David and Rachel.

SISTER ACT

WITH HER GROUP OF NEW-AGE NUNS, A CALIFORNIA WOMAN IS ON A MARIJUANA MISSION OF MERCY.

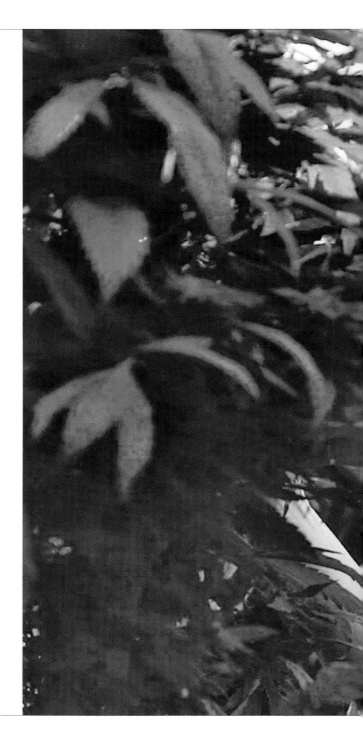

There was a time in her life when Christine Meeusen was convinced there was something inherently bad about marijuana. In fact, when she was around 20, she went to her future (and later ex) husband's apartment and saw his roommate cleaning cannabis stems and seeds off the kitchen table. And she panicked.

"I remember running into his bedroom, locking the door, and calling him at work because I was so afraid his roommate was going to rape me," she says. "That's what I thought of people with cannabis. It's the most ridiculous thing in the world now, though, as I look back on that moment."

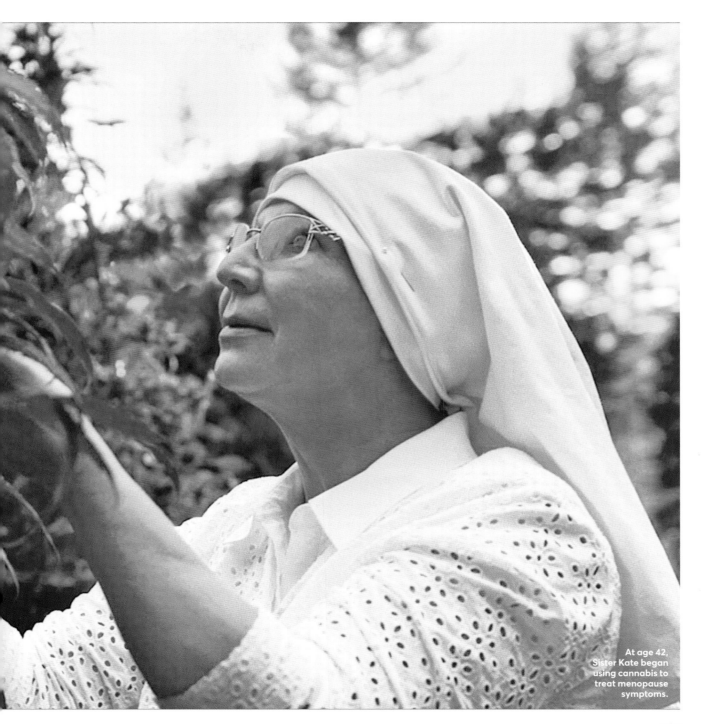

At age 42, Sister Kate began using cannabis to treat menopause symptoms.

That's because circumstances have definitely changed. First, she's no longer known as Christine Meeusen. She's called Sister Kate and lives in Merced County, California, where she operates a cannabis farm that's providing medicinal marijuana for patients around the world courtesy of her nondenominational spiritual group known as Sisters of the Valley. The divorced former marketing consultant and mother of two took up an interest in social activism in 2011 after she thought she'd heard Congress had declared pizza was a vegetable (actually, it was conservative representatives who insisted the tomato paste on pizza should qualify it as a vegetable to skirt school lunch requirements). Meeusen decided that "if pizza is a vegetable then I'm a nun" and, after being dared to dress as a nun for an Occupy Wall Street protest she attended, she was branded "Sister Occupy" by reporters. Sister Kate was born.

That led to her launching her makeshift "convent," making her first batch of cannabis in 2014 and starting Sisters of the Valley in 2015 as part of her "mission to help people empower themselves." These days, Sisters of the Valley has grown to include 23 "brothers and sisters," all of whom work together to make and sell nearly $1 million a year of THC-free CBD medicines, in everything from salves to tinctures to soaps. Some live on the 1-acre farm Sister Kate operates in Merced County, while others live a few hours north on her additional one-acre grow. Although her order is most definitely not a Catholic one, those who join her do takes vows of service and activism.

Not everyone is a fan of Sisters of the Valley, who were featured in the documentary *Breaking Habits*, which premiered at the Cannes Film Festival in early 2019. Sister Kate has had to battle both local law enforcement and thieves who came after her cannabis, as well as bankers who have tried to shut down her business. We spoke with her to learn more about her worldwide fan club, the lives she's saved and her plans for a Sisters of the Valley cartoon show.

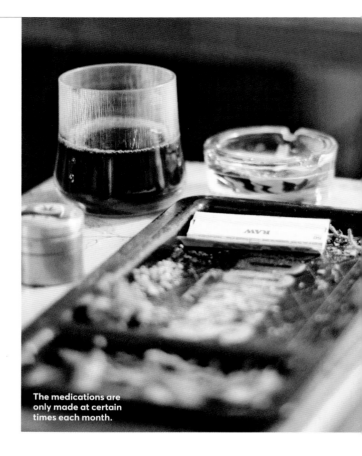

The medications are only made at certain times each month.

Even though you have all the trappings of a religious order, you're nondenominational. Has that ever gotten you in trouble with organized religions?

That's actually been the most shocking thing since I started Sisters of the Valley. I didn't think people would be upset about us covering our head [with habits] and saying this is our belief system. I honestly thought it would be the cannabis plant that would cause more problems, so it's been shocking to me that people were pissed off about our order. It's totally turned around, however. We've actually gotten gift boxes from nuns in another state, filled with trinkets from other convents. We told one of those sisters that

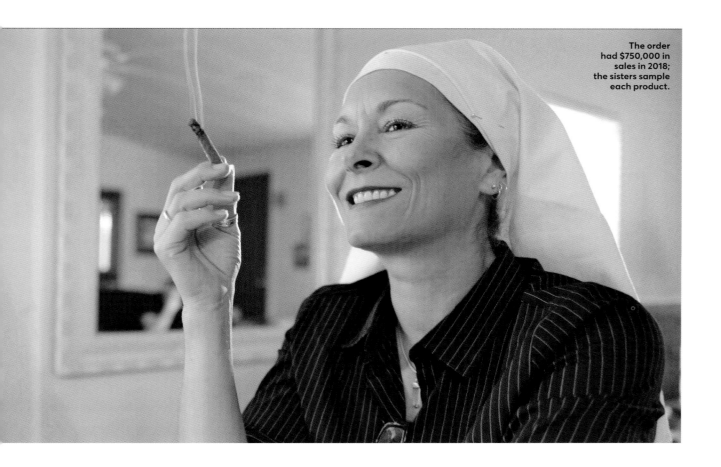

we wanted to send them any product of ours and asked what they would like. They wrote back and said, "Send seeds please!"

What is the biggest challenge that you have had to contend with?

Well, we lost our banking, so there have been challenges there. I took it personally. In the teaser for the documentary, the local sheriff says that we're doing this because we just want to get high. The day after that was shown, we got a letter from the bank saying we couldn't run any transactions through our account anymore. So now we're in our seventh week

keeping our store open but having no access to our funds, although I think we're finally on the cusp of solving the problem. It's been tough, though. All our sisters had to cash in savings and retirement plans to pay their bills. Many of our brothers and sisters are a check away from not making their mortgages.

You've persevered for several years now. Do you think you're slowly finding more acceptance wtihin the community?

I've joked that I have to get into the cocaine business now because it's getting too quiet here. We went to the state fair the other day, and we were like celebrities!

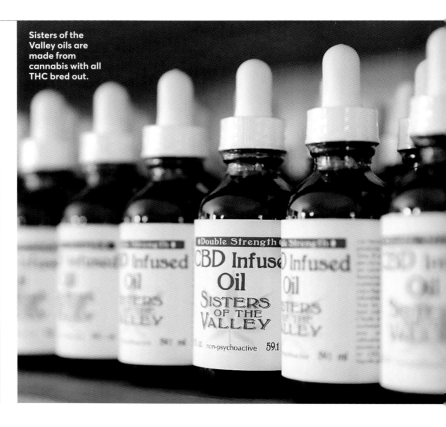

Sisters of the Valley oils are made from cannabis with all THC bred out.

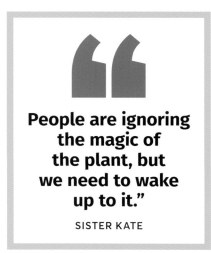

> **People are ignoring the magic of the plant, but we need to wake up to it."**
>
> SISTER KATE

Even the people from the sheriff's office were nice to me. There was a concert with Morris Day and the Time and the security guard asked if we'd like to go backstage and meet the band, even though I didn't know who they were. Sister Alice and Sister Sierra and I even danced onstage in front of 5,000 people!

Cannabis has made you like rock stars now!
Ha! Well, we are collaborating on a number of projects with Emil Nava, who directed Ed Sheeran's first video, I think. He sends a film crew whenever we're out on a political venture. But something I really want to do is a sort of "Sisters of South Park" cartoon series. We've spent the past few years saving up our best little bits for it. It'd be something political, edgy, relevant, new...it's a project close to our hearts.

Do you ever hear any feedback from the people who are buying your medicine?
We see miracles here every week. There was one guy who swears he had a brain tumor and the only thing he did differently after the diagnosis was use our tincture for 90 straight days. And after that, he says, the tumor was nearly gone. We get stories like that all the time. There was a young girl in Bakersfield who was having 100 seizures a day. A sister heard about this and wrote the mother and sent a CBD gift package to encourage her to try it as treatment. That young sister moved on, and then I got a call from the mom saying, "I know you mean well, but these medicines are stacking up and there's no way I can give it to her." I told her, "Oh my God! What kind of mother are you that

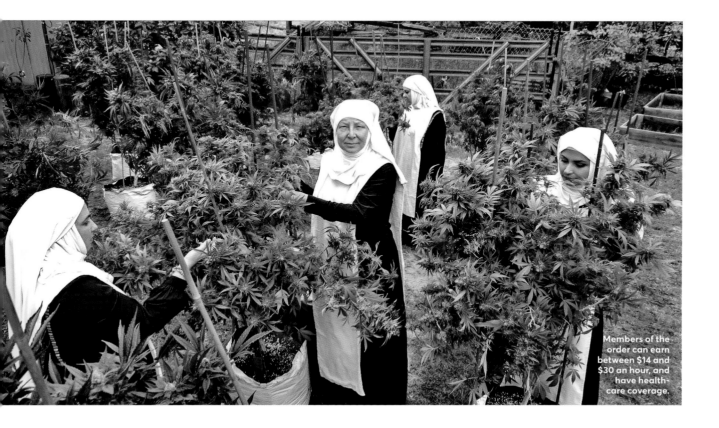

Members of the order can earn between $14 and $30 an hour, and have health-care coverage.

you won't experiment to help your own daughter?" I gave her hell, and she was nice about it. She now loves me for it.

CBD seems like it's everywhere these days. What sets your medicine apart from others?

We make it by using a combination of ancient wisdom and modern science. We start up making a batch on the new moon and complete it on the full moon. We also have a tribal celebration with every full moon, and during the two weeks we're making the medicine, we don't eat meat. The batches are also labeled with the moon's cycle. We do a prayer ceremony at the beginning of every batch. At the same time, though, we believe in science and use a lab to test all our products.

Where can people find your goods?

You can get more information on Sisters of the Valley products at sistersofcbd.com. We get orders from everywhere. We're selling in England and Canada, and hopefully in Mexico, when they decide what we can ship. Ultimately, we don't want the medicine to travel. We want what's purchased in Germany to be made in Germany. As we grow the order, we'll be able to close the gap for how far the medicine travels. Our goal is to sustain our farm operations and compassionate activism by making products for the people in a spiritual environment. At this point, we have 12 sisters globally who have taken the vows and about 10,000 people worldwide who have expressed an interest in joining the order. I've been busy and haven't done anything with that. Yet!

A

ACDC (Charlotte's Web), 52, 54, 144

Acupuncture, CBD-enhanced, 124

Addiction, cannabis use and, 59, 126-127

Age/Aging, cannabis use and, 60, 110-113

Ailments. See Conditions/diseases; specific ailments, conditions, and diseases

Alzheimer's disease, 67

American Cannabinoid Clinics (ACC), 176-179

American Medical Association (AMA), 128

American Refugee Foundation (AMRF), 175

Americans for Safe Access (ASA), 17

Anandamide (CB1 receptor), 19-21

Anorexia, 67

Anxiety reduction, CBD use for, 30, 35, 67, 69

Appetite, cannabis use and, 59-60

Athletic recovery, 73

Autism, cannabis oils and, 173

B

Back pain, 68, 86-90

Barry, Rick, interview with, 148-151

Belushi, Jim, interview with, 152-157

Blue Dragon Desert Frost, 54

Books, on medical cannabis, 101

Brain, THC and CB1/CB2 receptors and, 21-23

Brain tumor, personal healing experience, 166-169

Breaking Habits (documentary), 182

Brown, Mary, 66

C

Cancer
cannabis for symptom relief in, 92-95
chemotherapy side-effects, cannabis alleviating, 96-97
personal healing experiences, 96-97, 132-134, 136-137, 173

Cannabinoids. See also CBD (cannabidiol); CBG (cannabigerol); THC (tetrahydrocannabinol)
for inducing sleepiness, 80-83
receptors. See CB1 receptor; CB2 receptor

Cannabis, medical use of. See Medical cannabis/marijuana

Cannabis caregivers, 118-121

Cannabis oil. See also CBD oils
for marijuana massage, 125
personal healing experience with, 105, 165, 173, 175

Cannabis pain patches, 41

Cannabis sativa, 20, 26
CBD extraction from, 26
growing, 49, 52, 141. See also Growers

CannaKids, 166, 167, 168, 173

Capsules, CBD, 29

Card, medical marijuana, 46-49

Caregivers, cannabis, 118-121

CB1 receptors, 19-21
CBD interaction with, 22, 26, 28

CB2 receptors, 19-21
CBD interaction with, 22, 26, 28
pain relief and, 68, 76, 77

CBD (cannabidiol), 8

acupuncture and, 124
in cannabis, 37
extraction from cannabis flowers, 26
in hemp, 26
limits of, 128-129
THC partnership with, 20-21, 38
use in pets, 114-117

CBD oils, 88, 163, 184
differences between, 128
personal healing experience, 144, 171
use with pets, 116
vaping with, 29

CBD products, 24-25
broad-spectrum, 28
choosing between, 35
dosing advice, 28, 30-31, 35
evaluating source of, 31
medical benefits, 28
tips on selecting, 32-35
ways to consume, 29

CBD:THC (equal ratio) tincture, 39

CBG (cannabigerol), 67, 68, 73, 74, 77, 78, 97

Charlotte's Web (ACDC), 52, 54, 144

Chasen, Emma, 66

Chem 4, 54

Chemotherapy side-effects, cannabis alleviating, 96-97

Chicken pox, 78

Children, cannabis use in
for debilitating conditions, 78, 79
personal healing experiences, 166-175

Chong, Tommy, 132-134, 136-137

Clifton, Dr. Mary, 66

Common cold, 60-61, 68

Conditions/diseases
healing power of cannabis in, 64-79. See also specific ailments, conditions, and diseases
qualifying, for medical marijuana card, 48, 49
Consumption methods, 35, 38-41. See also specific methods
Corazon, 54
Cost
of medical marijuana card, 48, 157
per dried ounce of marijuana, 49
"Craft hemp," 35, 128
Crohn's disease, 68
facts about, 172
personal healing experience, 170-172

D

Debilitating conditions, in children, 78, 79
Declassifying cannabis, Dr. Oz on, 162-164
Delivery systems. See Consumption methods
Depression, cannabis use in, 68, 81
personal healing experience, 98-101
Detectability, in body system, 127
Diabetes, 68
Dispensary(ies)
cannabis caregivers and, 120
establishing trust in, 34
locating, 48
medical marijuana card and, 47-49
operating procedures, 56
recreational, 49

Doctors. See Physicians
Dopamine, THC and CB1 receptors activation in brain, 22, 23
Dosido, 54
Dosing advice/guidelines, 28, 30-31, 35, 36-41, 58, 140
for pets, 116, 117
sleep and, 82-84
Dravet syndrome, personal healing experience, 174-175
Drescher, Fran, interview with, 138-141
Dry-herb vaping, CBD, 29
Dynasty Electrik duo, 124

E

ECS (Endocannabinoid system), 16, 18-21
Edibles, 35, 40
dosing calendar for, 40
pet treats, 116
Elderly, cannabis use and, 60, 110-113
Endocannabinoid system (ECS), 18-21
acupuncture and, 124
Epidiolex, 70
Epilepsy. See Dravet syndrome; Seizures
Etheridge, Melissa, 135
Exercise, cannabis use and, 58-59

F

Falling asleep
terpenes and, 71, 76
tips for, 81
Farm Bill (2018), 26
Fibromyalgia, 70
Figi, Charlotte, 52, 144, 145, 147. See also ACDC (Charlotte's Web)

Flu, 60-61, 70
Fox, Michael J., 135
Fragile X syndrome, 78
Freeman, Morgan, 135

G

"Gateway drug," 129
Generations, conversation between, 7
Glaucoma, 70, 71
Glioma, optic nerve, personal healing experience, 166-169
Goldberg, Whoopi, 135
Goldstein, Dr. Bonni, 66
Growers, 52, 163
Belushi Farm, 152-157
Danny Sloat, 98-101
Sisters of the Valley, 180-185
Growing cannabis, for own use, 49
Gummies, CBD, 29
Gupta, Dr. Sanjay, 23, 52
interview with, 142-147
Gynecomastia, 128

H

Hard drugs, 129. See also Opioids
Healing properties, of cannabis, 64-79. See also specific ailments, conditions, and diseases
Hemp
legalization of, 26
products, 35
Hepatitis, 71
High CBD:Low THC tincture, 39
High THC:Low CBD tincture, 39
Holistic healing, cannabis enhancement of, 122-125

I

ID (medical marijuana card), 46-49

Illness, healing power of cannabis in, 64-79. *See also* specific ailments, conditions, and diseases
Immune system, cannabis use and, 60-61
    modulating response, 68, 70, 76
Incredibles (medical-cannabis company), 175
Ingestion method
    benefits of, 68
    CBD products, 35, 39-40
Inhalation methods, vaping vs. smoking, 38-39, 61
Insomnia, 81, 84
Insomnia relief, 35, 71, 76
Insurance coverage, 48

J
Jock itch, 73

K
Kidney disease, 73
Knox, Dr. Rachel
    on cannabis for cancer symptom relief, 94-95
    interview with, 56-61
Knox family physicians, interview with, 176-179

L
Labeling, CBD products, 34-35
Lady Gaga, 135
Legal issues, 17
    medical marijuana card and, 49
Legalization
    cannabis
    Mehmet Oz on, 164-165
    Sanjay Gupta on, 23
    hemp, 26

public support for, 7-8
Lemmiwinks, 54
LSD (marijuana strain), 54
Lupus, 73

M
Marijuana, medical uses for. *See* Medical cannabis/marijuana
Massage, marijuana, 125
Maui Bubble Gift, 55
Medical cannabis/marijuana
    books on, 101
    dosing guidelines, 36-41
    Mehmet Oz on, 158-165
    Sanjay Gupta on, 23, 52, 142-147
    effects of, 16
    Fran Drescher's experience with, 138-141
    growers. *See* Growers
    Jim Belushi on, 152-157
    legal issues and, 17, 49. *See also* Legalization|
    physicians and, 42-45
    pros and cons of, 12-16
    Rick Barry on, 148-151
    strains of, 48, 50-55
    Tommy Chong's experience with, 132-134, 136-137
    uses for, 16
Medical marijuana card, 46-49
Medicating methods, 35, 38-41. *See also* specific methods
Meeusen, Cristine (Sister Kate). *See* Sisters of the Valley
Memory loss, cannabis use and, 127-128
Menstrual cramps, 73
Migraines, 73
Military war veteran, personal healing experience, 108-109
Mironchik-Frankenberg,

Elizabeth, DVM, on CBD for pets, 116, 117
Multiple sclerosis, 73
Muscle relaxation, 30
Myths, about marijuana, 126-129

N
Nasal strays, CBD, 29
Nausea, 74
New-age nuns. *See* Sisters of the Valley

O
Obesity, 74, 75
Oils. *See* Cannabis oil; CBD oil
Old age, cannabis use in, 60, 110-113
Opioids, cannabis as alternative to, 102-105
    Mehmet Oz on, 160, 162
    Sanjay Gupta on, 144, 147
Optic nerve glioma, personal healing experience, 166-169
Overdosing, 41, 128
Oz, Dr. Mehmet, 158-165

P
Pain relief
    cannabis patches, 41
    CB2 receptors and, 68, 76, 77
    CBD products for, 35
    Mehmet Oz on, 160-162
    Sanjay Gupta on, 144, 147
    opioids vs. cannabis for, 102-103
    personal healing experiences, 86-90, 98-101
    Rick Barry on, 148-151
Parkinson's disease, 74
Pediatric patients. *See* Children, cannabis use in
Pew Research Center, 7

Physicians, medical marijuana and, 42-45, 48, 56
  Knox family, interview with, 176-179
Phytocannabinoids, 18-21, 58, 61, 124. See also CBD (cannabidiol)
Pills, CBD, 29
Pineapple Jager, 55
Platinum Tiger Cookies, 55
Possession, amounts allowed, 49
Pre-rolls, CBD, 29
Prescribing vs. recommending marijuana, 48, 56
"Progress chart," from ASA, 17
Psoriasis, 74
Psychotropic compound. See THC (tetrahydrocannabinol)
PTSD (post-traumatic stress disorder)
  cannabis use and, 106-109
  CBD products for, 35
Pure CBD tincture, 39

Q
Q fever, 76

R
Recommending vs. prescribing marijuana, 48, 56
Reefer Madness (documentary), 7, 90, 126, 144
Rheumatoid arthritis, 76
Ringo's Gift, 55
Ryan, Tracy (founder of Canna-Kids), 166-167169

S
Seizures, 70
  Sanjay Gupta on, 144-145
  personal healing experience, 174-175

Sex life, cannabis use and, 59, 126
Sexual assault, personal healing experience after, 106-107
Shingles, 78
Sickness, healing power of cannabis in, 64-79. See also specific ailments, conditions, and diseases
Sister Wife, 55
Sisters of the Valley (new-age nuns), 180-185
Sleep. See Insomnia; Insomnia relief
Sleep disorders, 82
Sleep hygiene, 84
Sloat, Danny (cannabis grower), personal healing experience, 98-101
Smoking, vaping vs., 38-39, 61
Snoop's Dream, 55
Sound therapy, cannabis-enhanced, 124
Sports recovery, 73
Stewart, Patrick, 135
Strains, marijuana, 48, 50-55
Strawberry Satori, 55
Stroke, 76

T
Terpenes, 52, 97
  in combination with CBD, 68
  falling asleep and, 71, 76
  in marijuana, 162
  non-cannabinoid, 82
THC (tetrahydrocannabinol), 8, 18
  in cannabis, 37
  CB1 receptor and, 21-23
  CB2 receptor and, 21-23
  CBD partnership with, 20-21, 38
  CBD-THC ratios in tinctures, 39

endocannabinoid system and, 20
  in hemp, 26
  overdosing, 41
Tikun Olam (cannabis research firm), 31
Tinctures, CBD, 29
  types of, 39
Topicals, 29
  dosing guidelines, 41
Tourette's syndrome, 77
Traumatic experiences, cannabis use following, 106-109

U
Ulcerative colitis, 77

V
Vape pen experiences, 89-90, 156
Vaping CBD, 29
  smoking vs., 38-39, 61
Vascular disease, 78
Vendors, 31, 34. See also Dispensary(ies)

W
Wasting syndrome, 78
Weight reduction, cannabis use and, 59
Williams, Montel, 160, 162
Workouts, cannabis use and, 58-59

Y
Yeast infection, 78
Yoga, cannabis-enhanced, 124-125

Z
Zoster viral infection, 78

Cover Emilija Randjelovic/Getty Images; underworld/Shutterstock **2-3** bortonia/Getty Images **4-5** Norman Posselt/Getty Images **6-7** George Peters/Getty Images **8-9** Visual Generation/Shutterstock **10-11** belterz/Getty Images **12-13** content_creator/Shutterstock **14-15** rgbstudio/Alamy **17** VICTOR DE SCHWANBERG/Getty Images **18-19** Prostock-Studio/Getty Images; MOLEKUUL/Getty Images **20-21** Lifestyle Discover/Shutterstock **22-23** SEBASTIAN KAULITZKI/Getty Images; MOLEKUUL/Getty Images **24-25** Clockwise from top left: Smith Collection/Getty Images; Columbia Pictures/Everett Collection; Denver Post/Getty Images; CQ-Roll Call/Getty Images; NurPhoto/Getty Images; Oleg Zharsky/Stocksy **27** Creative-Family/Getty Images **29** Clockwise from top right: ballyscanlon/Getty Images; Bill Diodato/Getty Images; Giada Canu/Getty Images; Tiny Ivan/Alamy; IRA_EVVA/Shutterstock; Artem Hvozdkov/Getty Images **30-31** CucuMberStudio/Shutterstock **32-33** Nodar Chernishev/Getty Images **34** Tinnakorn jorruang/Shutterstock **35** Foodio/Shutterstock **36-41** George Peters/ Getty Images (4) **43** Creative Family/Shutterstock **44-45** Kanjana Kawfang/Shutterstock **46-47** Aleynikov Pavel/ Shutterstock **48-49** calvindexter/Getty Images **50-51** SunnyToys/Shutterstock **52-53** NinaM/Shutterstock **54-55** Justin McIvor/Lochfoot (14) **57** paulynn/Shutterstock **58-59** Martin Novak/Getty Images; Lauren Burke/Getty Images **60** ImagePixel/Getty Images **61-62** GeorgePeters/Getty Images **65** CSA-Printstock/Getty Images **66** Brenda Rose/Getty Images **66-79** CSA-Printstock/Getty Images (7) **80-81** LaylaBird/Getty Images **83** Caitlin Riley/Getty Images **84-85** LaylaBird/Getty Images **86-87** Image Source/Getty Images **89** HighGradeRoots/Getty Images **90-91** Tetra Images/Alamy **92-93** Sebastian Ervasti/Getty Images **95** YelenaYemchuk/Getty Images **102-103** subjob/Getty Images **104-105** IRA_EVVA/Getty Images **106** martin-dm/Getty Images **110-111** MStudioImages/Getty Images **112** manonallard/Getty Images **115** Aleksandr_Kravtsov/Getty Images **116** Jonathan Weiss/ Alamy; rgbspace/Getty Images **118-119** H_Ko/Shutterstock **121** karacheo/Shutterstock **122-123** Clockwise from top left: da-kuk/Getty Images; Stevica Mrdja/Getty Images; Thom Lang/Getty Images; PeopleImages/Getty Images; Microgen/Shutterstock; KarinaUrmantseva/Getty Images; Microgen/Shutterstock **125** Westend61/ Getty Images **126** Kelly/Getty Images **127** Dennis Galante/Getty Images **128-129** PeopleImages/Getty Images **130** GeorgePeters/Getty Images **134** Jason LaVeris/Getty Images **135** Clockwise from top left: Neilson Barnard/ Getty Images; Getty Images for AARP; Jason Szenes/Shutterstock; Vittorio Zunino Celotto/Getty Images; Kevin Winter/Getty Images; Charles Sykes/Getty Images **141** Stephen Lovekin/Shutterstock **142-143** Noel Vasquez/ Getty Images **146-147** Brennan Linsley/AP Photo **148-149** Matrosov/Getty Images **150** Focus On Sport/Getty Images **151** Steve Jennings/Getty Images **152-157** Tyler Maddox (6) **158** David McNew/Getty Images **159,161** NBC/Getty Images (2) **162** Eugene Gologursky/Getty Images **163** Helen H. Richardson/Getty Images; Mitch M/Shutterstock **164** The Washington Post/Getty Images **165** CQ-Roll Call/Getty Images **166** Leah Moriyama **168** info@jencastlephotography.com **176-177** ElRoi/Shutterstock **180-185** Good Deed Entertainment (5) Back Cover underworld/Shutterstock

SPECIAL THANKS TO CONTRIBUTING WRITERS

Tess Barker, Steve Bloom, Joanna Cachapero, Tom Cunneff, Alan Di Perna, Joe Dolce, Anne Driscoll, Nicola Farris, Sabrina Ford, Lisa Greissinger, Erik Himmelsbach-Weinstein, Nicole Pajer, Maria Speidel, Irene Zutell

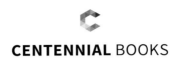

CENTENNIAL BOOKS

An Imprint of
Centennial Media, LLC
40 Worth St., 10th Floor
New York, NY 10013, U.S.A.

ISBN 978-1-951274-26-9

Distributed by
Simon & Schuster, Inc.
1230 Avenue of the Americas
New York, NY 10020, U.S.A.

For information about custom editions, special sales and premium and corporate purchases,
please contact Centennial Media at contact@centennialmedia.com.

Manufactured in China